NEURODEGENERATIVE DISEASES -
LABORATORY AND CLINICAL RESEARCH

MOLECULAR MECHANISMS INVOLVED IN THE PATHOGENESIS OF HUNTINGTON'S DISEASE

NEURODEGENERATIVE DISEASES - LABORATORY AND CLINICAL RESEARCH

Additional books in this series can be found on Nova's website under the Series tab.

Additional E-books in this series can be found on Nova's website under the E-book tab.

NEURODEGENERATIVE DISEASES -
LABORATORY AND CLINICAL RESEARCH

MOLECULAR MECHANISMS INVOLVED IN THE PATHOGENESIS OF HUNTINGTON'S DISEASE

CLAUDIA PERANDONES
FEDERICO EDUARDO MICHELI
AND
MARTÍN RADRIZZANI

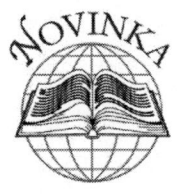

Nova Science Publishers, Inc.
New York

Copyright © 2010 by Nova Science Publishers, Inc.

All rights reserved. No part of this book may be reproduced, stored in a retrieval system or transmitted in any form or by any means: electronic, electrostatic, magnetic, tape, mechanical photocopying, recording or otherwise without the written permission of the Publisher.

For permission to use material from this book please contact us:
Telephone 631-231-7269; Fax 631-231-8175
Web Site: http://www.novapublishers.com

NOTICE TO THE READER
The Publisher has taken reasonable care in the preparation of this book, but makes no expressed or implied warranty of any kind and assumes no responsibility for any errors or omissions. No liability is assumed for incidental or consequential damages in connection with or arising out of information contained in this book. The Publisher shall not be liable for any special, consequential, or exemplary damages resulting, in whole or in part, from the readers' use of, or reliance upon, this material.
Independent verification should be sought for any data, advice or recommendations contained in this book. In addition, no responsibility is assumed by the publisher for any injury and/or damage to persons or property arising from any methods, products, instructions, ideas or otherwise contained in this publication.
This publication is designed to provide accurate and authoritative information with regard to the subject matter covered herein. It is sold with the clear understanding that the Publisher is not engaged in rendering legal or any other professional services. If legal or any other expert assistance is required, the services of a competent person should be sought. FROM A DECLARATION OF PARTICIPANTS JOINTLY ADOPTED BY A COMMITTEE OF THE AMERICAN BAR ASSOCIATION AND A COMMITTEE OF PUBLISHERS.

LIBRARY OF CONGRESS CATALOGING-IN-PUBLICATION DATA

Available upon Request
ISBN: 978-1-61728-971-2

Published by Nova Science Publishers, Inc. † New York

Contents

Preface		vii
Chapter 1	Huntington's Disease	1
Chapter 2	Molecular Pathogenesis of Huntington'S Disease	23
Chapter 3	Conclusion	37
References		39
Index		51

PREFACE

Huntington's disease (HD) is an autosomal-dominant, progressive neurodegenerative disorder with a distinct phenotype, including chorea, incoordination, cognitive decline, and behavioral difficulties. The underlying genetic defect responsible for the disease is the expansion of a CAG repeat in the gene coding for the HD protein, huntingtin (htt). This CAG repeat is an unstable triplet repeat DNA sequence, and its length is inversely correlated with the age at onset of the disease. Expanded CAG repeats have been found in 8 other inherited neurodegenerative diseases. Despite its widespread distribution, mutant htt causes selective neurodegeneration, which occurs preferentially and most prominently in the striatum and deeper layers of the cortex.

Remarkable progress has been made since the discovery of HD gene in 1993. Animal models to study the disease process, unraveling the expression and function of wild-type and mutant huntingtin (htt) proteins in the central and peripheral nervous systems, and understanding expanded CAG repeat containing mutant htt protein interactions with CNS proteins in the disease process have been developed htt may cause toxicity via a wide range of different mechanisms. The primary consequence of the mutation is to confer a toxic gain of function on the mutant protein and this may be modified by certain normal activities that are impaired by the mutation. It is likely that the toxicity of mutant htt is only revealed after a series of cleavage events leading to the production of N-terminal huntingtin fragment(s) containing the expanded polyglutamine tract. Although aggregation of the mutant protein is the hallmark of the disease, the role of aggregation is complex and the arguments for protective roles of inclusions are discussed. HD progression has been found to involve several pathomechanisms, including expanded CAG repeat protein interaction with other CNS proteins, transcriptional dysregulation, calcium dyshomeostasis, defective mitochondrial bioenergetics and abnormal vesicle trafficking. Notably, not all the effects of mutant htt are cell-autonomous, and it is possible that abnormalities in neighboring neurons and glia may also have an impact on connected cells.

The present review focuses on HD, outlining the effects of mutant htt in the nucleus and cytoplasm as well as the role of cell-cell interactions in the HD pathology. The widespread expression and localization of mutant htt and its interactions with a variety of proteins suggest that mutant htt engaged multiple pathogenic pathways. A better understanding of these mechanisms will lead to the development of more effective therapeutic targets.

Chapter 1

HUNTINGTON'S DISEASE

1.1. INTRODUCTION: UNSTABLE EXPANDING REPEATS AS A NOVEL CAUSE OF DISEASE

Prior to this decade, the adage of "like-begets-like" fitted nicely with the dogma of human genetics where the genetic material was considered stable upon transmission and in the rare instance of mutation, the new variant itself was stably inherited. Although there had been clear instances when this didn´t hold true, the human genetics community did not embrace the notion of "dynamic mutations".

Clinical researchers had long suspected something was amiss when carefully examining families with dominant Myotonic Dystrophy where to find that off-springs of affected individuals often had a more severe form of the disease.

The term "anticipation" was used to define this progressive increase in expressivity of the identical mutation over a number of generations.

Since anticipation did not easily fit with the biological dogma of the genetics of that era, the concept of anticipation was summarily dismissed as an ascertainment bias. Many years later, the recognition of increasing penetrance through subsequent generations in Fragile X syndrome, subsequently known as the Sherman Paradox, resembled the genetic anticipation of Myotonic Dystrophy.

While the observation in Fragile X syndrome was more easily accepted by the scientific community, the Sherman paradox, like anticipation, could not be readily explained at a molecular level.

Provided it´s true, the phenomenon, represents one of the darkest black boxes in molecular genetics.

In 1991, the genes responsible for the Fragile X syndrome and Spinobulbar Muscular Atrophy were found to contain unstable, expanded trinucleotide repeats. The following year, Myotonic Dystrophy was also found to be the result of an expanded trinucleotide repeat. These findings were soon followed by a remarkable number of neurological disorders, each sharing the mutational mechanism of the unstable expansion of a repeat, most often being a triplet in form.

Soon, the behavior of these repeats in affected families clearly revealed a pattern where the increasing penetrance (Sherman Paradox) or increasing expressivity (Anticipation) through subsequent generations correlated with increasing lengths of the triplet repeat. Thus, a biological basis of anticipation, the dynamic mutation, was defined.

1.2. COMMON FEATURES OF DISEASES DUE TO UNSTABLE EXPANDING REPEATS

Trinucleotide repeat expansions now account for at least 16 neurological disorders ranging from childhood developmental disorders such as X-linked mental retardation syndromes to the late onset neurodegenerative disorders such as Huntington disease and the inherited ataxias. The variability in repeat size underlies the broad spectrum of phenotypes seen in each of these disorders. The repeats show somatic and germline instability. Successive generations of families affected by such dynamic mutations experience anticipation or earlier age of onset and more rapid disease progression owing to intergenerational repeat instability. For example, the onset of Myotonic Dystrophy ranges from birth in children and grandchildren to adulthood in parents and grandparents, depending on the size of the repeat.

Although unstable trinucleotide are the most common repeats to cause neurological disorders, others,such as tetra-and pentanucleotides expand to cause type 2 Myotonic Dystrophy and Spinocerebellar Ataxia type 10, respectively.

Several developmental and neuromuscular disorders are caused by either an insertion or a duplication of a small trinucleotide repeat (GCG)n typically encoding alanine. Examples of such disorders include hand-foot-genital syndrome, synpolydactyly, oculopharyngeal muscular dystrophy, and the X-linked mental retardation caused by mutation in the Aristaless-related homeobox gene (*Brais et al., 1998, Stromme et al., 2002, Utsch et al., 2002*).

These disorders differ from the classic trinucleotide expansion disorders because the expansions are small and are not as dynamic.

Tables 1, 2 and 3, provide a concise description of these disorders, the mutational basis, gene product, and key clinical features. The disorders have been divided according to pathogenic mechanism, i.e., whether mutations cause loss of function of the protein or gain of function of the RNA or protein or cause a yet-to-be-determined mechanism.

The expanded triplet repeats can be found in transcribed RNA destined to be untranslated (either 5´ or 3´ such as in fragile X syndrome or Myotonic Dystrophy, respectively), spliced out intronic sequence (such as in Friedreich´s Ataxia), or coding exonic sequence (such as the dominant ataxias) (Figure 1). In general, the noncoding repeats are able to undergo massive expansions from a normal number of 6-40 triplets to an abnormal range of many hundreds or thousands of repeats. This leads to either transcriptional suppression, as in the case of Fragile X syndrome, or abnormal RNA processing, limiting the amount of mature cytoplasmic message, as in the case of Myotonic Dystrophy. In contrast, the coding expansions undergo much more modest expansions from a normal range of approximately 10-35 repeats to an abnormal range of approximately 40 to 90 triplets. Since these are CAG repeats coding for polyglutamine tracts, constraints of the individual protein structures significantly modify this range. This is most apparent in SCA 6 where the largest normal allele contains 18 repeats whereas the smallest abnormal allele contains 21 repeats. In all coding expansions, the mechanism(s), while still poorly understood, appear to reflect a gain or change of function of the abnormal protein, eventually leading to neurodegeneration.

Common features of the diseases caused by expansion of an unstable CAG repeat within a gene include:

- They are all late-onset neurodegenerative diseases, and except for Kennedy disease, are all dominantly inherited.
- The expanded allele is transcribed and translated.
- The trinucleotide repeat encodes a polyglutamine tract in the protein.
- There is a critical threshold repeat size, below which the repeat is nonpathogenic and above which it causes disease.
- The larger the repeat above the threshold, the earlier the age of onset (on average; predictions cannot be made for individual patients, but there is a clear statistical correlation).

- The CAG repeat disease genes so far identified are widely expressed and encode proteins of unknown function. When the polyglutamine tract exceeds the threshold length, the protein aggregates, forming an inclusion body that apparently kills the cell.
- The different clinical features of each disease reflect killing of different cells, presumably because of interactions with other cell-specific proteins.
- Neuronal cell death caused by protein aggregates is a common thread in the pathology of CAG repeat diseases, Alzheimer disease, Parkinson disease and prion diseases; the mechanism and their general significance remain to be discovered.

1.3. Clinical and Genetic Aspects of HD

In 1872, Dr. George Huntington published a seminal work title "On Chorea". This manuscript described the features of an illness observed among the members of three families residing in East Hampton, New York. Dr. Huntington called the disease "hereditary chorea" and his observation on the mode of inheritance is remarkable because the basic tenants of genetics, as defined by Gregor Mendel, had not been recognized at this time. Dr. Huntington described the transmission of the disease in the following terms: "When either or both of the parents have shown manifestations of the disease... one or more of the offspring almost invariably suffer from the disease, if they live to adult age. But if by any chance these children go through life without it, the thread is broken and the grandchildren and great-grand children of the original shakers may rest assured that they are free from the disease". This description provides a functional description for the autosomal dominant mode of transmission with complete penetrance characteristic of HD.

Dr. Huntington's treatise was of such clarity that it was reprinted in prominent neurology texts and termed "Huntington's Chorea". More recently, the observation that some cases, and particularly those with a young onset, may present without chorea, has led to the widespread adoption of the designation Huntington's Disease (HD) to refer to this affliction.

Huntington's Disease

Location of trinucleotide expansions in humans

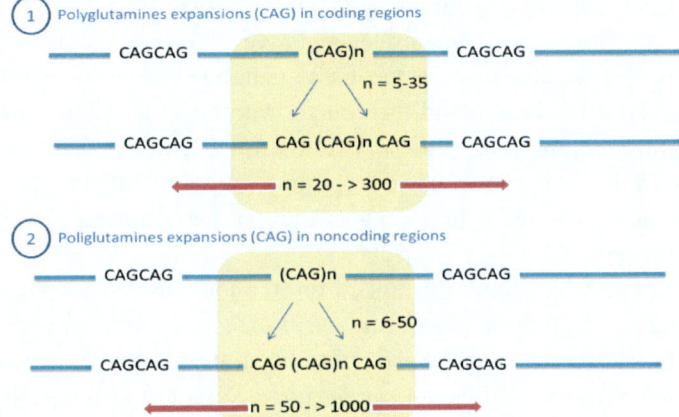

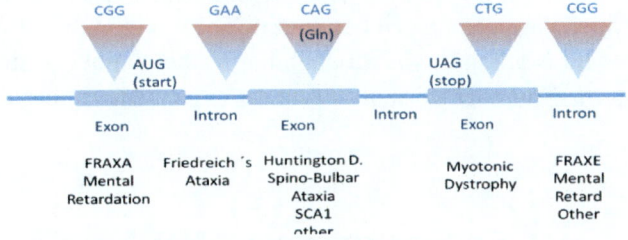

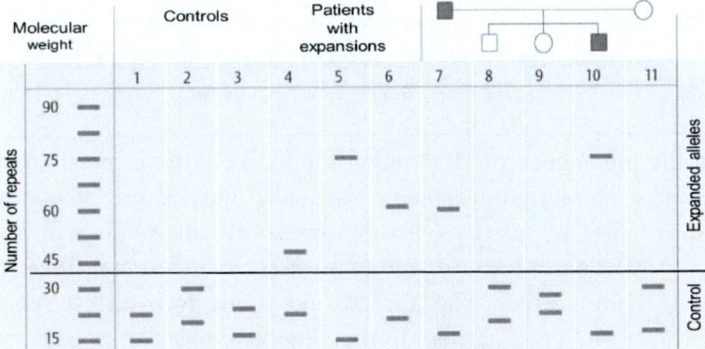

Panel 1. Polyglutamine (CAG) expansions in coding regions
Panel 2. Polyglutamine (CAG) expansions in noncoding regions
Panel 3. Different locations of trinucleotide expansions
Panel 4. Laboratory diagnosis of trinucleotide repeat disorders

Figure 1. Location of trinucleotide expansions in humans.

HD is a midlife-onset disease which strikes at a mean age of 40 years, but onset may vary from 4 to 80 years of age (Harper, 1992).

It is a progressive neurodegenerative disorder with primary neuropathological involvement in the basal ganglia. HD is invariably fatal, without periods of remission, and the course from onset to death averages 15 to 17 years (*Myers, Sax et al. 1991*). The disease is characterized mainly by involuntary choreiform movements, cognitive impairment, and personality disorder featuring to depression, anger and temper outbursts, as well as cognitive disorders.

The HD gene was genetically linked to an anonymous marker located in 4p16.3 (Figure 2) (*Gusella, Wexler et al. 1983*) and, following a 10-year molecular genetic search, was discovered to be an unstable CAG trinucleotide repeat (*The Huntington's Disease Collaborative Research Group, 1993*). The mutation extends a polymorphic stretch of CAG codons in the first exon of the HD gene, lengthening a segment of polyglutamine near the amino terminus of the HD protein which has been named huntingtin. The mutation which leads to the expression of HD is an approximate doubling in the number of the triplet repeats from a normal number of about 18 to an expanded number of 40 or more.

1.4. Epidemiology of HD

The prevalence of HD is estimated at 5 to 10 affected persons per 100,000 among individuals of European descent but is less common among other ethnic groups (*Harper, 1992; Al-Jader, Harper et al., 2001; Bertram and Tanzi, 2005*).

Indeed, the prevalence of HD among the native African population is so low as to make an accurate estimate difficult, and its prevalence among Japanese and Asian populations is approximately one-tenth that the one observed in Caucasians. Because, for each affected individual, there are an estimated two living carriers who are still too young to manifest symptoms, the prevalence of HD gene carriers in the general Caucasian population may be estimated at 15 to 30 per 100,000, and there are an equal number of at risk siblings who are the ones who have not inherited the HD defect. Thus, approximately 1 in every 2500 births is an individual born at risk for the disease, making HD the most common of the CAG repeat expansion diseases.

Table 1. Unstable repeat disorders caused by loss-of-function, RNA mediated, or unknown mechanisms

A. Loss of function mechanism

Disease	MIM number	Repeat Unit	Gene Product	Normal Repeat	Expanded Repeat	Main clinical features length
FRAXA	309550	(CGC)n	FMRP	6-60	>200 (full mutation)	Mental retardation, macroorchidism, connective tissue defects, behavioral abnormalities
FRAXE	309548	(CCG)n	FMR2	4-39	200-900	Mental retardation
FRDA	229300	(GAA)n	Frataxin	6-32	200-1700	Sensory ataxia, cardiomyopathy, diabetes.

B. RNA-mediated pathogenesis

Disease	MIM number	Repeat Unit	Gene Product	Normal Repeat	Expanded Repeat	Main clinical features length
DM1	160900	(CTG)n	DMPK	5-37	50-10.000	Myotonia, weakness, cardiac conduction defects, insulin resistance, cataracts, testicular atrophy, and mental retardation in congenital form
DM2	602668	(CCTG)n	ZNF9	10-26	75-11.000	Similar to a DM1 but no congenital form
FXTAS	309550	(CGG)n	FMR1 RNA	6-60	60-200	Ataxia, tremor, Parkinsonism and dementia.

A. Disorders produced by a loss of function mechanism
B. Disorders produced by RNA-mediated pathogenesis.

Table 2. Unstable repeat disorders caused by unknown pathogenic mechanisms

Disease	MIM number	Repeat Unit	Gene Product	Normal Repeat	Expanded Repeat	Main clinical features length
SCA 8	608768	(CTG)n	SCA 8 RNA	16-34	>74	Ataxia, slurred speech, nistagmus.
SCA 10	603516	(ATTCT)n		10-20	500-4500	Ataxia, tremor, dementia.
SCA 12	604326	(CAG)n	PPP2R2B	7-45	55-78	Ataxia and seizures
EHL2	606438	(CTG)n	Junctophilin	7-28	66-78	Similar to HD.

Table 3. Polyglutamine disorders caused by gain-of-function mechanisms

Disease	MIM number	Gene Product	Normal Repeat	Expanded Repeat	Main clinical features length
Huntington disease	143100	Huntingtin	6-34	36-121	Chorea, dystonia, cognitive deficits, psychiatric problems.
SCA 1	164400	Ataxin 1	6-44	39-82	Ataxia, slurred speech, spasticity, cognitive impairments.
SCA 2	183090	Ataxin 2	15-24	32-200	Ataxia, polyneuropathy, decreased reflexes, infantile variant with retinopathy.
SCA 3	109150	Ataxin 3	13-36	61-84	Ataxia, parkinsonism, spasticity.
SCA 6	183086	CACNA1a	4-19	10-33	Ataxia, disarthria, nistagmus, tremors.
SCA7	164500	Ataxin 7	4-35	37-306	Ataxia, blindness, cardiac failure in infantile form.
SCA 17	607136	TBP	25-42	47-63	Ataxia, cognitive decline, seizures, and psychiatric problems.
SBMA	313200	Androgen Receptor	9-36	38-62	Motor weakness, swallowing, gynecomastia, decreased fertility.
DRPLA	125370	Atrophin	7-34	49-88	Ataxia, seizures, choreoathetosis, dementia.

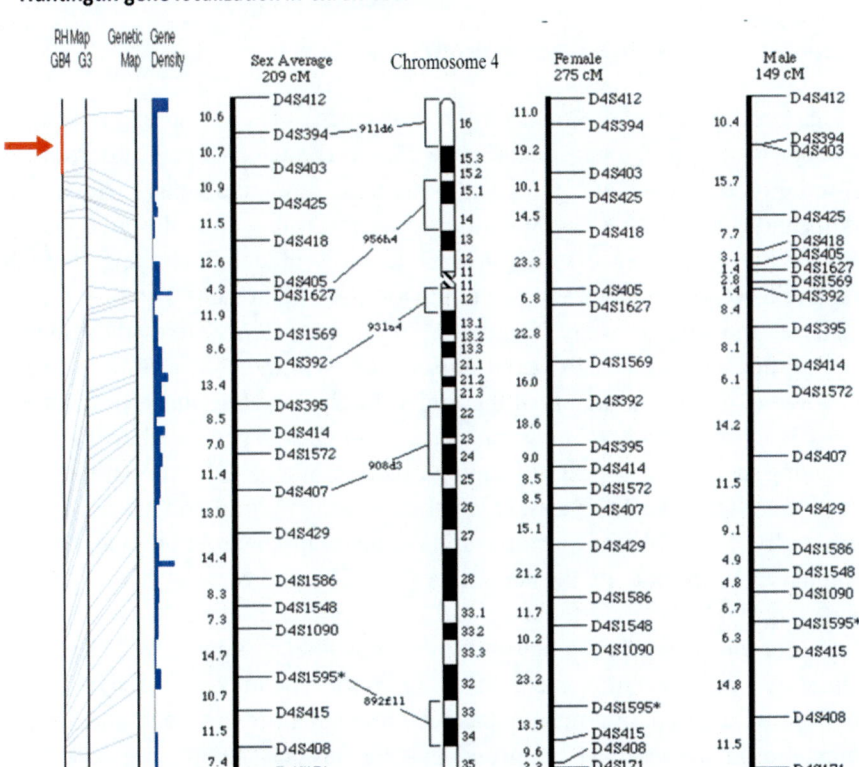

The cytogenetic bands of the short arm of chromosome 4 (4p) are depicted with the location of the HD defect in 4p16.3 from genetic linkage and physical mapping studies indicated. The map of 4p16.3 provides an expanded view of this telomeric cytogenetic band to illustrate the location of the defect relative to polymorphic DNA markers used to sequentially narrow the minimal HD genetic region by recombination analysis, linkage disequilibrium, and haplotype analysis.

Figure 2. Huntingtin gene localization in Chromosome 4.

Genotype-phenotype correlations in HD, therefore, most likely will allow the description of uncommon events such as new mutations or alleles with reduced penetrance which may be too rare to be observed in other triplet repeat diseases.

1.5. CLINICAL CORRELATES IN HD

A. Chorea and Motor Impairment

The term chorea is of Greek origin and means dance. Chorea refers to a prominent feature of the gait disturbance characteristic of HD and the "dance-like" quality of movement. Choreic movements are involuntary, slow, and random and may involve any voluntary muscle group. Thus the involuntary aspect of the movement disorder in HD features random twitching of both upper and lower extremities and of both the left and right sides.

These movements may begin as mild myoclonic like movements involving the fingers, toes, or facial muscles early in the course of the disease and evolve to large movements of the limbs and trunk as the illness progresses. Progressively, movements may interfere with gait, speech, chewing, and swallowing, and other aspects of motor function associated with activities of daily living. However, the extent of the movement impairment may vary substantially for different persons and some may have little evidence of involuntary movement. In the late stages of HD, chorea may lessen and is replaced by rigidity and dystonia.

In addition to the involuntary choreic movement impairment, there is a slowing of voluntary movement. This bradykinesia may be seen in tasks involving rapid alternating movements, eye movements and finger, and tongue tapping. Some studies have proposed that the progression of impairment in involuntary movements may be more uniform across different stages of HD and may therefore represent a more consistently progressing feature for assessments of disease course than the severity of chorea.

The relation of motor impairment to CAG repeat size has not been widely studied. Andrew et al. (*Andrew, Goldberg et al.1993*) found no association between the repeat length and the form of clinical presentation (e.g., motor, mood, or cognitive disturbance as the initial feature).

B. Age at Onset

The age at onset of HD is highly variable. The earliest cases have been reported with onset at 2 to 3 years of age while the latest onsets approach 80 years or even older. The average is at age 40 and is not sex related. Approximately 7% of all cases present before the age of 20 and this group of individuals has traditionally been termed "juvenile" onset HD.

The impact of the HD repeat upon phenotypic expression has been heavily investigated. The relationship between age at onset and repeat size is unequivocal and very strong but it is not linear; most investigators have noted that the best fit is a model in which the repeat predicts the log10 of onset age (*Ranen, Stine, et al. 1995*). For the 220 HD cases depicted in Figure 3, the correlation between repeat size and log of onset age is r = - 0.84 and accounts for about 70% of the variance in onset age.

Kremer et al (*Kremer, Squitieri, et al. 1993*), noted that for late-onset cases, with onset at age 50 or older, the correlation of onset with repeat size is reduced (r=-0.29).

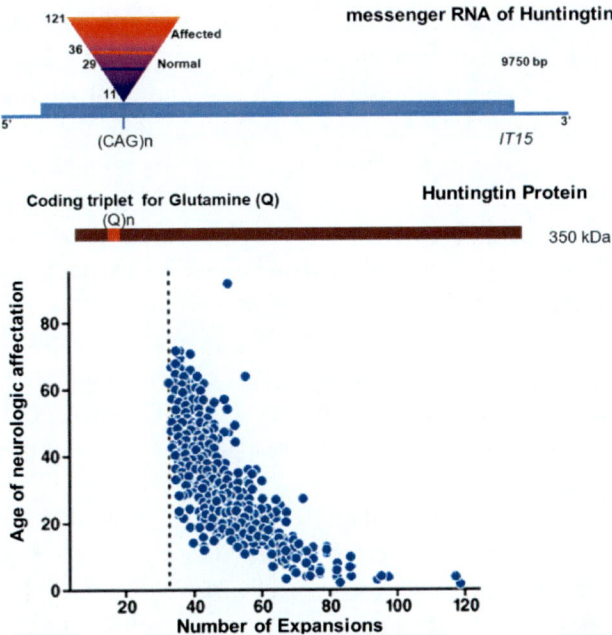

Relationship between the length of the expanded HD CAG repeat and age at neurological onset of disease. The CAG repeat sizes for 220 individuals affected with HD diagnosed through the New England Huntington's Disease Research Center are presented in relationship to the age at onset of motor impairment. Repeat size is strongly related to age at onset. Onset age before age 20 is usually associated with a repeat size of more than 60 CAG units. Among persons with adult onset, the range in onset age for a given repeat is large and may vary by 35 years or more.

Figure 3. Relationship between length of CAG repeat and age at neurologic onset of disease.

It has been noted that there is a +- 18-year 95% confidence interval around the estimated onset age for a given repeat size. Although one group recently suggested that the confidence interval may be smaller than this estimate, all published reports confirm that the range in onset age for a given repeat size exceeds 30 years among persons with mid- and late-life disease.

Thus, for more than 90% of presymptomatic HD cases the relationship of repeat size is not strong enough to predict the onset age.

C. Rate of Disease Progression

The course of disease in HD is remarkably variable, but there have been only a few studies of factors related to progression (*Myers, Sax, et al. 1991*). There is evidence that age at onset is related to rate of progression and it has been proposed that a single mechanism influences both the age at onset and the rate of disease progression. Although not strong enough to predict onset pre-symptomatically, the HD repeat size appears to be the primary determinant of onset age and thus it is reasonable to expect that the repeat size is related to the rate of disease progression as mediated either by its effect upon onset age or by a direct effect upon disease progression.

A study of a set of monozygotic twins reared apart suggested that progression is largely determined by genetic factors and the most likely determinant is the trinucleotide repeat size (*Sudarsky, Myers, et al., 1983*).

Many authors have reported a significant association between repeat size and rate of disease progression.

Another factor is the sex of the affected parent, with offspring of affected fathers having a more rapid progression than offspring of affected mothers. In addition, lower body mass index early in the disease is related to more rapid disease progression.

While the sex of the affected parent and paternal transmission is now known to be related to the transmission of an expanded repeat, it is not known whether the repeat size influences weight loss or lower body mass index (*Marder, Zhao H, et al. 2009*).

These studies are relevant when considering trials for therapeutic interventions which will need to consider the HD repeat in the randomization of study participants.

D. Neuropsychology

1. Cognitive Function in HD

While language functioning remains relatively intact, the most striking cognitive deficits involve areas of executive system functioning (e.g., strategies in problem solving and cognitive flexibility), short-term memory, and visuospatial performance. The memory disorder is characterized by inconsistent retrieval of information. In the early stages of the disease, recognition memory for verbal information is robust, while spontaneous recall of information may be more frequently impaired.

Early in the disease process the cognitive deficits are relatively focal. A global, progressive subcortical dementia does not evolve until the disease advances significantly. Although this dementia is significant and debilitating in the late and final stages of the disease, it is qualitatively different from the cortical dementia observed in Alzheimer's disease (*Duff, Beglinger, et al. 2009*).

2. CAG Relationship to Cognition

Andrew et al. (*Andrew, Goldberg, et al. 1993*) found no association between the CAG repeat length and the form of clinical presentation (e.g. motor, mood, or cognitive disturbance as the initial feature) and others have also failed to find a relationship between the repeat length and either the type of symptom onset or disease progression or the type of psychiatric involvement. However, these observations seem to be valid only for early or mid-life age onset cases of the disease. A retrospective observational study of thirty-four persons with late onset of Huntington Disease (HD) (onset range 60-79 years) performed by Lipe and Bird (*Lipe and Bird, 2009*) showed that when CAG trinucleotide expansion size ranged from 38-44 repeats, motor problems were the initial symptoms at onset.

Many works have tried to established correlations between cognitive functions and different parameters of progression or severity in HD.

Peinemann et al. (*Peinemann, Sabine, et al. 2005*) conducted a study which aim was to clarify if cognitive dysfunction in early stages of HD is correlated with loco-regional structural changes in 3D-MRI. HD patients demonstrated robust regional decreases of gray matter volumes in the caudate and the putamen. Executive dysfunction was significantly correlated with the areas of highest significant differences out of voxel-based morphometry (VBM) results which were located bilaterally in the caudate. Moreover, subgroup analyses revealed marked insular atrophy in HD patients who performed worse in the single executive tasks.

Two aspects were most remarkable in this correlational study: (i) striatal atrophy in HD patients in early stages plays an important role not only in impaired motor control but also in executive dysfunction, and (ii) extrastriatal cortical areas, i.e., the insular lobe, seem to be involved in executive dysfunction as assessed by neuropsychological tests requiring for planning and problem solving, stimulus response selectivity and concept formation.

E. Clinical Correlates of Mitochondrial Function in HD Muscle

Mitochondrial function analyses on HD postmortem brain demonstrated a severe defect of mitochondrial complex II/III activity in the striatum. Studies have also shown abnormal bioenergy in the HD brain in vivo, with elevated lactate and reduced N-acetyl aspartate within the striatum. Htt expression is not restricted to the CNS and has been documented in skeletal muscle and myoblast cultures from the R6/2 transgenic mouse model of HD.

Many studies reported a defect of mitochondrial ATP synthesis capacity in HD skeletal muscle in vivo, which correlated inversely with the length of the CAG repeat i.e. the longer the repeat, the worse the defect (*Lodi R, Schapira AH, Manners D, et al. 2000*). Furthermore, gene expression profiles of R6/2 HD transgenic mice and HD skeletal muscle have also demonstrated changes with a transition from fast to slow-twitch fibers in the mutants, suggesting an adaptive response to muscle that is less dependent on oxidative phosphorylation (*Strand, Aragaki, et al. 2005*).

The study of Turner et al. (*Turner, Cooper, et al. 2007*) demonstrated that individual HD skeletal muscle complex II/III activity correlated with clinical disease progression and with the cognitive score on the Unified HD Rating Scale (UHDRS), two measures of functional status, the age of the patient, disease duration and the repeats years score.

The reduction in the complex II/III function showed a strong correlation with disease progression on several clinical scales independently of an age-related phenomenon.

It seems possible that a progressive reduction in complex II/III activity occurs in HD patient muscle and this could cause a sequence of biochemical events that may include damage, as is proposed for HD striatum.

Mitochondrial dysfunction and specifically complex II/III activity might be involved in the sequence of HD pathogenesis and this can be correlated with worsening of many clinical parameters. Prolonged treatment with free radical scavengers may ameliorate the progressive loss of complex II/III activity and modify disease progression.

1.6. ISOLATION OF THE HD MUTATION

The clinical and genetic characteristics of HD, including its distinct symptoms, midlife onset, unambiguous mode of inheritance, high penetrance, and prevalence in the general population, made it an ideal disease to approach using strategies based on genetic linkage. In 1983 the HD defect was mapped to the vicinity of an anonymous polymorphic DNA marker, D4S10, following the inheritance of restriction fragment length polymorphisms in two large HD kindred, of American and Venezuelan descent (*Gusella, Wexler, et al. 1983*).

Genetic linkage to D4S10 established that virtually all cases of HD were likely to arise from defects in the same gene (*Conneally, Haines et al., 1989*). These early linkage studies also demonstrated that D4S10 was ~4cM (~4% recombination) from HD, providing the basis for the molecular diagnosis of HD in asymptomatic at-risk individuals able to participate in a genetic linkage test.

Linkage to D4S10 revealed the complete phenotypic dominance of HD. Affected homozygotes, possessing two copies of the HD defect, were discovered to be clinically indistinguishable from their heterozygous siblings with one copy of the mutation (*Wexler, Young et al., 1987; Myers, Leavitt et al., 1989*).

A consortium of investigators employed a combination of genetic and physical mapping techniques to confine the mutation to a segment of ~ 2 million base pairs of 4p16.3. Simultaneously, they generated genetic and physical maps of the region, developing overlapping clone sets, and refining the defect's location using recombination analysis in disease pedigrees and linkage disequilibrium between the disorder and genetic markers.

The location of the HD gene (Figure 2) was pinpointed ultimately by an analysis of haplotypes formed by multiallele markers from across the region which revealed that although ~two thirds of disease chromosomes had unrelated haplotypes and likely had independent origins, the remaining ~one third shared a small (275 kb) region between D4S95 y D4S180. This provided strong evidence that this subset of disease chromosomes was likely to be descended from a common ancestral chromosome (*MacDonald, Novelleto et al., 1992*).

Analysis of candidate genes from this subregion finally led to the discovery of a polymorphic CAG repeat in the 5' end of interesting transcript 15 (IT15) that was expanded and unstable on disease chromosomes.

1.7. THE HD TRINUCLEOTIDE REPEAT MUTATION

The pure stretch of CAG trinucleotide repeat that is expanded on disease chromosomes is located near the 5' end of a novel 4p16.3 gene (Figures 1 and 7), immediately adjacent to a broken array of CAG/CCG codons containing a mildly polymorphic (6 a 12 repeats), stably transmitted stretch of CCG triplets.

The results of initial genotype-phenotype correlation studies quickly revealed that most normal chromosomes and the majority ($\geq 90\%$) of disease chromosomes possess 7 CCG repeats (*Rubinztein, Barton, et al., 1993*), whereas the adjacent array of pure CAG repeats was found to be highly polymorphic. Normal chromosomes possessed from 6 to 34 CAG repeats that are inherited in a Mendelian fashion and HD chromosomes from 39 to ~ 86 units that are inherited in a strikingly non-Mendelian manner. Moreover, rare alleles with 36-39 repeats were found in exceptional individuals, the unaffected elderly relatives of sporadic de novo cases of the disease.

These initial findings made it possible to offer a direct DNA test, Polymerase Chain Reaction (PCR) amplification determination of the HD CAG repeat length, to many at risk individuals in a wide variety of testing situations. The findings of subsequent genotype-phenotype studies performed in research and clinical diagnostic laboratories around the world have provided critical data for the generation of testable hypotheses for the mechanism of action of the HD mutation. These results provided evidence, for example, that the length of CAG repeat in the expanded range is strongly correlated with the age at onset of the disease, with age at onset decreasing as the CAG repeat size increases (Figure 3: Relationship between length of CAG repeat and age at neurologic onset of disease).

They also pointed out that any given expanded CAG repeat is associated with a broad range of onset ages, highlighting the relevance of other factors in determining age at onset in any single individual.

Currently four CAG repeat size intervals are recognized as associated with varying disease risk in HD (Figure 4: Repeat size and HD risk).

These ranges have been defined by the U.S. H.D. Genetic Testing Group (USHDGTG) and are derived from information gleaned from more than 1000 HD tests. Nevertheless, the disease-related risk corresponding to the 29 to 39 repeats range is often based upon fewer than 10 observations at each repeat size, and thus, these risk estimates can be expected to change with additional information.

a) Normal: repeat sizes up to 26 units

Individuals with repeats in this range do not develop HD, nor has there been a confirmed instance of a child inheriting HD from a parent with a repeat in this range.

b) Nonpenetrant with paternal meiotic instability: repeats of 27 to 35 units.

Repeats in this range are rare and represent approximately 1% of expanded alleles seen in HD testing protocols. There have been no confirmed reports of persons with repeats in this range expressing HD. There are, however, confirmed cases of paternally transmitted meiotic instability such that descendants of fathers with repeats in this range are known to have inherited an expanded allele in the clinical range. There are no reported cases of maternally transmitted meiotic instability in this range, producing offspring with repeats in the clinical range (*Semaka, Creighton, et al. 2006*).

c) Reduced penetrance with meiotic instability: Repeats of 36 to 39 units

Repeats in this range are rare and represent approximately 1 to 2% of expanded alleles seen in HD testing programs. Some persons with repeats in this range develop HD and others live into their 90s without evidence of the disease (*Myers, MacDonald et al., 1993; McNeil, Novelleto et al., 1997*). There is clear evidence that penetrance increases with increasing allele size in this range. Penetrance has been roughly estimated at 25 % for 36 repeats, 50% at 37 repeats, 75 % at 38 repeats, and 90 % at 39 repeats based upon USHDGTG data.

d) HD: Repeats of 40 units or larger

It is currently believed that all persons with repeats in the range of 40 or more will eventually develop HD.

However, some individuals with repeats at the low end of this range are reported to exhibit initial symptoms at ages older than common life expectancy and, thus, there may be some reduced penetrance among carriers of 40 or 41 repeats (*Brinkman, Mezei et al., 1997*).

Kenney et al (*Kenney, Powel, et al., 2007*) reported an autopsy proven HD case with 29 trinucleotide repeats. The patient presented with HD classic phenomenology and a great number of potential HD phenocopies with overlapping features have been excluded.

However, despite having performed additional histochemical staining, the authors failed to detect the presence of htt in the ubiquitin-positive neuronal intranuclear inclusions. Although the detection of the htt stain is not absolutely necessary to establish the neuropathological diagnosis of HD (*Jean Paul Vonsattel, MD, personal communication*) in this arguable case it would be relevant to confirm the presence or absence of the "mutated" protein in the nucleus as the subcellular localization of mutant htt is critical for the pathology of HD.

In agreement with this report, many recent experimental findings are shifting the focus from the polyglutamine expanded tract to other domains of the protein for toxicity (*Zoghbi and Orr 2009*). In other words, the concept that toxicity is simply a result of an expanded toxic polyglutamine tract that might escape the cellular degradation and quality control machinery becomes less likely.

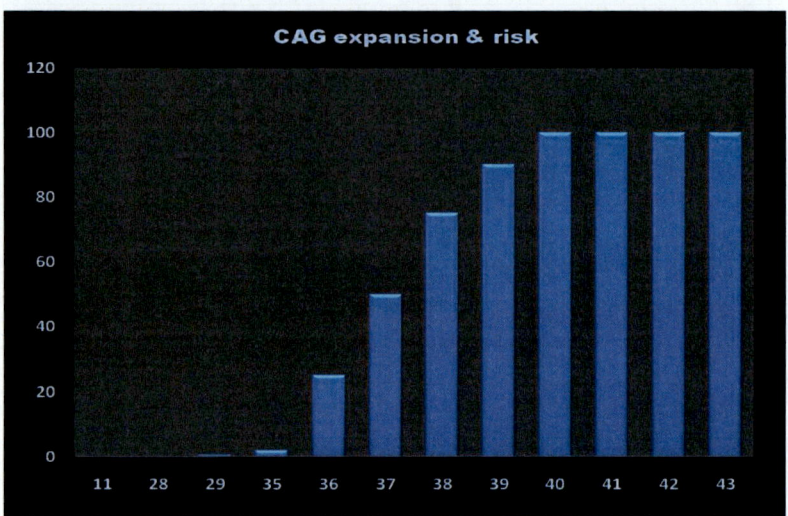

Four CAG repeat size intervals are recognized as associated with varying disease risk in HD. These ranges have been defined by the US HD genetic Testing Group (USHDGTG) and are derived from information gleaned from more than 1000 HD tests.

Figure 4. Repeat size and HD risk.

The expansions of the polyglutamine tracts although relevant, are not the only molecular mechanism to cause toxicity. Many studies in spinobulbar muscular atrophy and HD indicate that protein domains outside the polyglutamine tract play a significant role in the selective neurotoxicity observed in these diseases (*Graham, Deng et al., 2006*).

The fact that a repeat length of 29 CAG repeats can cause HD would significantly modify genetic counselling of HD families, HD therapeutic trials and the current understanding of the molecular pathogenesis of the disease.

1.8. NEUROPATHOLOGIC STUDIES IN HD

The brain regions initially affected in HD are the neocortex and the striatum, with the most extensive atrophy being demonstrated in these regions. The neurodegenerative process in the striatum occurs first in the caudate nucleus, than in the putamen (*Vonsattel and DiFiglia, 1998; Gutekunst, Norflus et al., 2000*). Pathological changes in the striatum develop in a seemingly topographically ordered manner, spreading along the caudal-rostral, dorsal-ventral and medial-lateral axes (Figure 5: Selective vulnerability of the striatum in HD).

The severity of post-mortem neuropathological features and cell loss have been graded using the scale described by Vonsattel, Meyers et al. 1985. HD pathology is divided into grades 0-4, designated in ascending order of severity. Neuropathological grade correlates with the severity of motor symptoms, mental state and CAG repeat length (*Rosenblatt, Abbott, et al. 2003*). Within affected brain regions, certain neurons degenerate whereas others remain relatively spared. In the striatum, medium spiny neurons which receive dense innervation from the cortex, are preferentially affected, with the sparser interneurons, lacking cortical innervations being relatively spared (*MacDonald and Halliday, 2002; Heinsen, Rub et al., 1999*). Most of these medium spiny neurons become dysfunctional and are eventually lost in HD, thus disrupting the circuitry of the basal ganglia.

Substantial degeneration also occurs in the cerebral cortex of patients with HD. Volume reductions are seen in associative, frontal, temporal, parietal and primary somatosensory cortices. Large cortical pyramidal neurons, including those that project directly to the striatum, are selectively lost. The disruption of corticostriatal circuitry in HD is known to contribute to the motor symptoms of the disease and may well also play a key role in cognitive symptoms.

Patients with HD have a heterogeneous presentation with regard to their clinical condition and progression, which may well reflect individual variations in patterns of neurodegeneration. For example, even in early to mid stages of the disease, structural magnetic resonance imaging (MRI) studies reveal that regions other than the neocortex and striatum, notably hippocampus, globus pallidus, amygdale and cerebellum, can also show morphometric changes (*Rosas, Koroshetz, et al., 2003*). Pathology in the neocortex and hippocampus may be of particular significance with regard to the cognitive deficits seen in HD.

Reactive microglia has been detected in the cortex and striatum of postmortem human HD brains. The density of activated microglia correlated with the degree of neuronal loss and Vonsattel grading. Markers of increased inflammatory gliosis have also been identified in the putamen and frontal cortex at post mortem and together, these findings suggest that an inflammatory process may be possibly contributing to HD, although it is not known whether this has any impact on disease onset or progression.

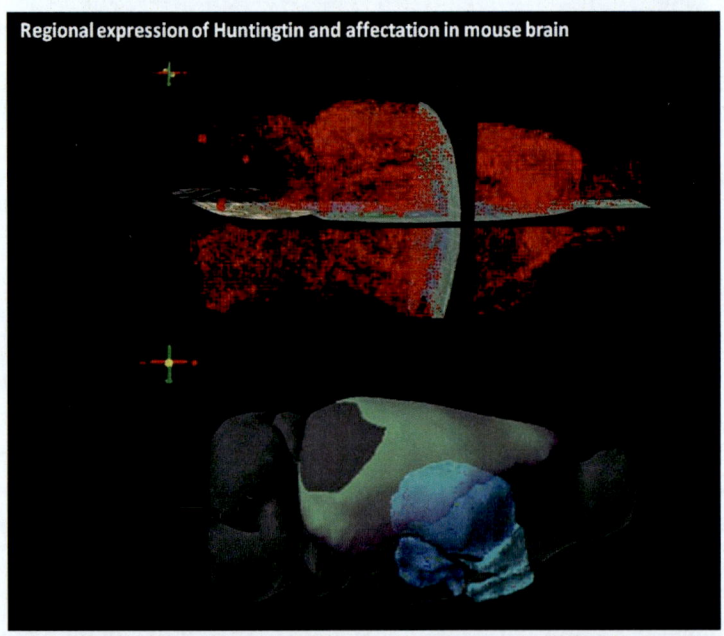

The genetic expression of Huntingtin can be observed through a tridimensional approach using "in situ hybridizations" performed with mRNAs in murine cerebral cortex slices (http://www.brain-map.org, Allen Institute for Brain Science. © 2004). The results of these hybridization assays are in concordance with the ones previously published in "Nature" (Site, Lein, E.S. et al., Genome-wide atlas of gene expression in the adult mouse brain, Nature 445: 168-176 (2007), doi:10.1038/nature05453). The bottom figure is a tridimensional reconstruction that highlights the regions that show selective vulnerability in HD, the striatum and cerebral cortex.

Figure 5. Selective vulnerability of the striatum in HD.

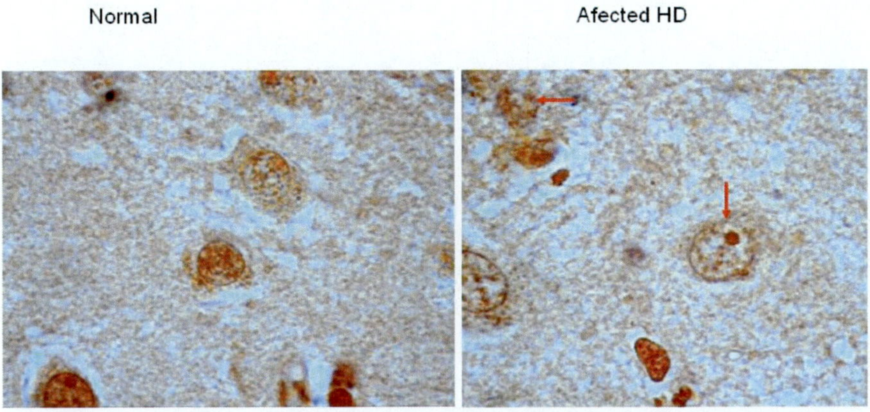

Normal   Afected HD

One characteristic neuropathological feature, present in both human HD patients and transgenic HD mice, is the presence of protein aggregates, also known as neuronal inclusions, which are formed from the aggregation of expanded polyglutamine-cointaining Htt fragments as well as numerous other proteins.

Figure 6. Neuritic aggregates and perinuclear inclusions in HD.

One characteristic neuropathological feature, present in both human HD patients and transgenic HD mice, is the presence of protein aggregates, also known as neuronal inclusions (Davies, Turmaine et al., 1997) (Figure 6: Neuritic aggregates and perinuclear inclusions in HD), which are formed from the aggregation of expanded polyglutamine-cointaining htt fragments as well as numerous other proteins.

The aggregates appear in many different tissues, including the cortex and the striatum, and can be seen in either the cell nucleus or the cytoplasm.

These protein aggregates appear to disrupt cytoskeletal structures closely associated with protein and mRNA trafficking to synapses, possibly leading to secondary deficits in synaptic signaling.

However, many evidences suggests that aggregates may represent a neuroprotective cellular strategy (*Menalled, Sison et al., 2003; Arrasate, Mitra et al., 2004*), with polyglutamine containing fragments possibly exerting their toxic effects on cellular processes such as gene expression and protein transport prior to the formation of the large aggregates visible using light microscopy (*Bodner, Outeiro et al., 2006; Bodner, Housman et al., 2006*).

Chapter 2

MOLECULAR PATHOGENESIS OF HUNTINGTON'S DISEASE

2.1. HD GENE AND GENE PRODUCT

The genetic defect responsible for HD is an expansion of a CAG repeat in the gene coding for the HD protein.This CAG repeat is an unstable triplet repeat DNA sequence, and its length is inversely correlated with the age at onset of disease, especially in juvenile HD cases, in which the repeat length is often >60 CAG units (*Andrew, Goldberg et al., 1993*) (Figure 7: A schematic diagram of human Huntingtin).

Expanded CAG repeats have been found in 10 other inherited neurodegenerative diseases, as well, including spinocerebellar ataxia (SCA) and spinobulbar muscular atrophy (SBMA) (*Zohbi and Orr, 2000; Gatchel and Zoghbi 2005; Butler and Bates 2006*) (see Tables 2 and 3). It is now clear that expansion of this repeat in various genes can cause distinct neurodegenerative pathology leading to different disorders.

The CAG repeat is translated into a polyglutamine (polyQ) domain in the disease proteins. Human htt is a large protein comprising 3144 amino acids. A normal polyQ domain, which in htt begins at amino acid position 18, typically contains 11-34 glutamine residues in unaffected individuals, but this expands to more than 37 glutamines in HD patients. The length of the polyQ repeat varies among species. For example, mouse htt has 7 glutamines, whereas pufferfish htt contains only 4 (*Harjes and Wanker 2003*), which suggests that the polyQ domain may not be essential, but that it can regulate protein function. Consistently, deletion of the CAG repeat in the HD gene only results in subtle behavioral and motor phenotypes in mice.

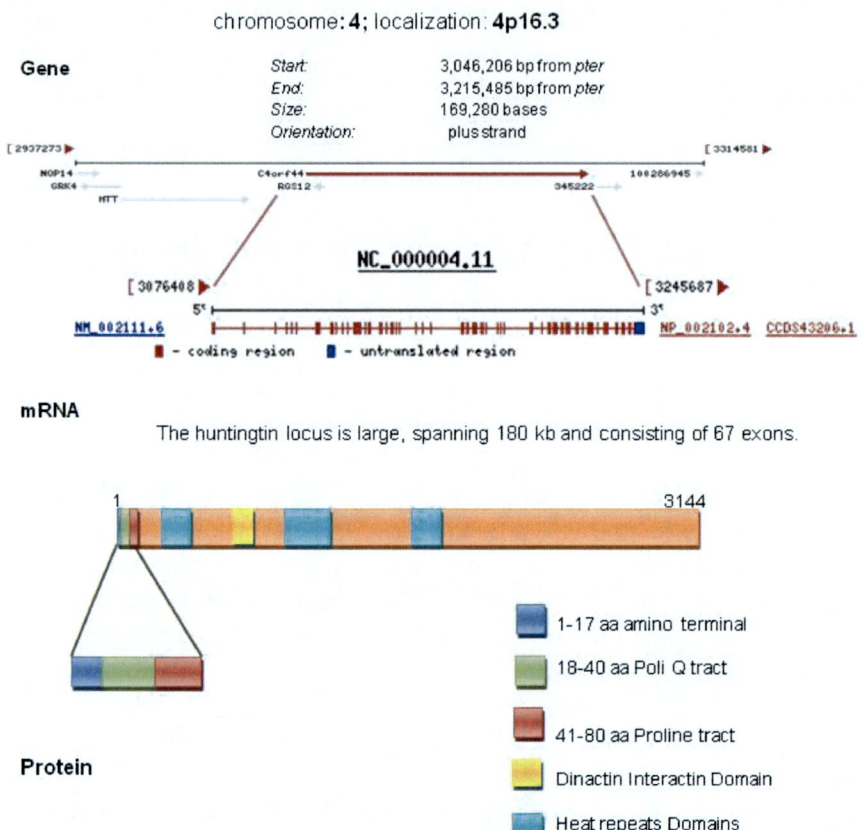

The diagram shows the structure of the gene, mRNA and htt protein.

Figure 7. A schematic diagram of human huntingtin.

Htt is ubiquitously expressed in the brain and body and distributed in various subcellular regions (*Gutenkunst, Levey et al., 1995*). Its sequences do not show homology to other proteins of known function. One structural feature of htt, is the presence of HEAT repeats (*Takano and Gusella 2002*), which are sequences of ~40 amino acids that occur several times within a given protein and are found in a variety of proteins involved in intracellular transport and chromosomal segregation (*Neuwald and Hirano 2000*).

Several lines of evidence also suggest that htt is involved in intracellular trafficking and various cellular functions. As an example, htt is associated with a number of subcellular organelles (*DiFiglia, Sapp et al., 1995; Gutekunst, Levey, et al., 1995; Sharp, Love et al., 1995; Gutekunst, Li et al., 1998*).

In concordance, htt is known to interact with a variety of proteins that can be grouped according to whether they are involved in gene transcription, intracellular signaling, trafficking endocytosis, or metabolism (*Harjes and Wanker 2003; Li and Li 2004*).

Identification of these htt-interacting proteins suggest that htt may function as a scaffold involved in coordinating sets of proteins for signaling processes and intracellular transport.

The essential role of htt has been established using HD gene knockout mice. In this model, the absence of htt causes cell degeneration and embryonic lethality (*Duyao, Auerbach et al., 1995; Nasir, Floresco et al., 1995; Zeitlin, Liu et al., 1995*). Conditional knockout mice also show degeneration in adult cells (*Dragatsis, Levine et al., 2000*). These observations have led to the theory that a loss of htt function may contribute to the neuropathology of HD (Loss of function hypothesis) (*Cattaneo, Rigamonti et al, 2001*). However, there is more evidence to support the theory wherein mutant htt gains a toxic function. (Gain of function hypothesis). For example, heterozygous HD knock mice are known to live normally. Further, identification of the HD gene has allowed the generation of various animal models in which mutant htt is expressed in the presence of endogenous normal htt, and these transgenic mice still develop neurological symptoms and die early, even when endogenous normal htt is expressed at the normal levels (*Davies, Turmaine et al., 1997; Schilling, Becher et al., 1999*).

Moreover, mutant htt can rescue the embryonic lethal phenotype of htt-null mice *(Hodgson, Smith et al., 1996)*, which also suggests the HD mutation can lead to neuronal toxicity, independent of the essential function of htt.

2.2. CORRELATION BETWEEN NEUROPATHOLOGY AND PATHOGENESIS IN HD

Despite its widespread expression, htt causes selective neurodegeneration, which occurs preferentially and most prominently in the striatum and deep layers of the cortex in the early stages of HD (*Vonsattel, Myers et al., 1985*). In advanced stages, other brain regions, such as the hippocampus, hypothalamus, cerebellum, amygdala, and some thalamic nuclei, are also affected. Among these other brain regions, the lateral tuberal nucleus of the hypothalamus exhibits severe atrophy (*Kremer, Roos et al., 1990*).

The neurons that are most severely affected in HD are striatal projection neurons, which send their axons to different brain regions. These are the GABAergic medium sized spiny neurons (MSNs), which constitute 95 % of all striatal neurons. MSNs receive abundant glutamatergic input from the cortex and primarily innervate the substantia nigra and globus pallidus. Thus, their preferential loss in HD is thought to be the result of glutamate excitotoxicity. Consistently, there is relative sparing of interneurons that colocalize somatostatin, neuropeptide Y, and NAPDH diaphorase, as well as of cholinergic interneurons and a subclass of GABAergic neurons that contain parvalbumin (*Ferrante, Kowall et al., 1985; Graveland, Williams et al., 1985; Vonsattel, Myers et al., 1985*). Another important pathological feature in the postmortem brains of HD patients is gliosis (*Myers, Vonsattel et al., 1991; Singhrao, Thomas et al., 1998; Sapp, Kegel et al., 2001*). Reactive glia or gliosis often occurs in response to neuronal injury. For example, neuronal degeneration is evidenced by a dramatic elevation in the density of large glia (*Rajkowska, Selemon et al., 1998*). Marked astrogliosis and microgliosis were observed in caudate and internal capsule samples of HD patients, but not in normal brain. In the striatum and cortex, reactive microglia also occurred in all grades of pathology, accumulated with increasing grade , and grew in density in relation to the degree of neuronal loss (*Ferrante, Kowall et al., 1985; Graveland, Williams et al., 1985; Vonsattel, Myers et al., 1985*). Thus, reactive microglia were considered to be an early response to change in neuropil (*Sapp, Kegel et al., 2001*). While reactive gliosis does represent an early neuropathological event in HD, glial pathology can also impact neuronal viability. Indeed, gliosis is a pathological feature in several HD mouse models that lack neuronal cell degeneration. These models include transgenic mice expressing N-terminal mutant htt (*Ishiguro, Yamada et al., 2001; Yu, Li et al., 2003; Gu, Li et al., 2005*) and "knock-in" mice that express full-length mutant htt (*Reddy, Williams et al., 1998; Lin, Tallaksen-Greene et al., 2001*).

Since the discovery of the HD gene, various antibodies and DNA aptamers against htt have been generated to characterize the distribution of mutant htt. Immunostaining of brains from transgenic mice that express mutant htt revealed nuclear inclusions (*Davies, Turmaine et al., 1997*). Similar nuclear inclusions were identified in the brains of HD patients (*DiFiglia, Sapp et al., 1997; Gutekunst, Li et al., 1999*). Subsequently, the accumulation of expanded polyQ-containing proteins in the nucleus and nuclear inclusions were found to be common pathological features of other polyglutamine diseases (*Zoghbi and Orr 2000; Gatchel and Zoghbi 2005; Butler and Bates 2006*). The role of these nuclear inclusions in HD remains controversial, since their formation is correlated with disease progression, but is not associated with neuronal degeneration (*Gutekunst, Li et al., 1999; Kuemmerle, Gutekunst et al., 1999; Slow, Graham et al., 2005*). Moreover, several studies have shown that htt inclusions are protective against htt toxicity in cultured cells (*Saudou, Finkbeiner et al., 1998; Arrasate, Mitra et al., 2004*). Despite the controversy surrounding their exact role, htt inclusions reflect protein misfolding caused by an expanded polyQ domain and represent a pathological hallmark for the accumulation of toxic mutant htt. It is also remarkable that normal htt is predominantly localized in the cytoplasm, whereas mutant htt with its expanded polyQ domain accumulates in the nucleus. Hence, nuclear inclusions reflect the aberrant accumulation of mutant htt in the nucleus.

Importantly, HD also features abundant cytoplasmic aggregates localized in neuronal processes (neuropil aggregates) including axons and dendrites (*Gutekunst, Li et al., 1999; Li, Li et al., 1999; Schilling, Becher et al., 1999; Li, Li et al., 2000; Li, Li et al., 2001; Menalled, Sison et al., 2003; Tallaksen-Greene, Crouse et al., 2005*). In the early stage of disease, the brains of HD patients contain more dystrophic neurites or neuropil aggregates than nuclear inclusions (*DiFiglia, Sapp et al., 1997; Gutekunst, Li et al., 1999*).

In addition, the progressive development of neuropil aggregates is strongly correlated with disease progression in transgenic mice (*Li and Li 1998; Li, Li et al., 1999; Li, Li et al., 2000; Li, Li et al., 2001*). Moreover, the neuropil aggregates are associated with axonal degeneration in HD mouse brains (*Li, Li et al., 2001; Yu, Li et al., 2003*).

Taken together, the localization of htt aggregates in the nucleus and neuronal processes reveals that mutant htt elicits toxicity in both the nucleus and cytoplasm.

2.3. MODELS FOR THE PATHOGENESIS OF HD

A number of mouse models have provided in vivo evidence for the pathology of HD. Several transgenic mice were generated using either the human htt promoter or neuronal promoters. For example, transgenic mice R6/2 express exon 1 htt with 115-150 glutamine repeats (115-150Q) under the control of the human HD gene promoter (*Davies, Turmaine et al., 1997*). YAC (Yeast Artificial Chromosomes) transgenic mice use the human HD gene promoter to drive the expression of full-length mutant htt (*Hodgson, Agopyan et al., 1999; Graham, Deng et al., 2006*). N171-82Q transgenic mice express the first 171 amino acids with 82Q under the neuronal prion promoter (*Schilling, Becher et al., 1999*). These transgenic mice have been widely studied and found to have neurological and behavioral phenotypes similar to those observed in HD patients.

There are also HD repeat knock-in mouse models, which are generated by inserting an expanded repeat into the endogenous mouse HD gene (*Shelbourne, Killeen et al., 1999; Wheeler, White et al., 2000; Lin, Tallaksen-Greene et al., 2001; Menalled, Sison et al., 2002*). However, most HD mouse models do not show the overt neurodegeneration seen in human HD patients, even though some models display severe neurological symptoms and early death (*Davies, Turmaine et al., 1997; Schilling, Becher et al., 1999*).

It is possible that the short life span of the mouse does not allow sufficient time for the development of obvious neurodegeneration, although some earlier pathological events do occur.

HD mouse models also suggest that small fragments containing expanded polyQ are more toxic than larger fragments (**HD and the toxic fragment hypothesis**). This fits with the finding that small N-terminal htt fragments are misfolded and form aggregates and inclusions in the brains of HD patients (*DiFiglia, Sapp et al., 1997; Gutekunst, Li et al., 1999*). It is obvious that proteolysis of htt generates multiple N-terminal htt fragments in HD repeat knock-in mice (*Zhou, Cao et al., 2003*). A great number of protease cleavage sites, including those for caspase-3, caspase-6, calpain, and unknown aspartic protease, have been found whithin the first 550 amino acids of htt (*Kim, Yi et al., 2001; Gafni and Ellerby 2002; Lunkes, Lindenberg et al., 2002; Wellington, Ellerby et al., 2002; Graham, Deng et al., 2006*).

In a recent study, the role of htt cleavage by caspase-3 and caspase-6 in disease was examined by expressing caspase-3 and caspase-6 resistant forms of mutant htt in mice. Controlling for expression levels, Graham, Deng et al., 2006, found that transgenic mice expressing polyglutamine-expanded htt with a mutated caspase-6 cleavage site did not manifest any behavioral deficits or neurodegeneration. In contrast, the caspase-3 resistant form of mutant htt remained fully pathogenic. Several assessments were performed to test the importance of the caspase-6 cleavage site in htt for disease. These included motor phenotypes (rotarod and open field) and neuropathology (brain weight, striatal volumen, and nuclear htt accumulation) of polyglutamine-expanded htt transgenic mice with a mutated cleavage site. Transgenic mice expressing polyglutamine expanded htt with a mutated caspase-6 cleavage site did not manifest behavioral deficits or neurodegeneration, even when the expression level of htt exceeded that of unmutated polyglutamine expanded htt transgenic mice. Also, htt mutated at caspase-6 cleavages sites had a significant delay in its nuclear translocation. Nuclear translocation is an early step in pathogenesis in a HD knock-in mouse model (*Wheeler, Gutekunst et al., 2002*) and is known to be required for neurotoxicity of other polyglutamine disease proteins.

These results demonstrate that sequences outside the polyglutamine tract are critical for pathogenicity and are consistent with cleavage of htt by caspase-6 as being a critical event for pathology in HD. However, the importance of caspase-6 cleavage for HD needs to be confirmed by manipulating caspase-6 activity in transgenic mice expressing full length mutant htt.

Most studies used transfected proteins to identified cleavage sites, and the nature of toxic N-terminal fragments generated organically in the HD brain is still being explored. It is likely that the proteolysis of full-length htt generates a number of N-terminal htt fragments. The decreased activities of the proteasomes and chaperones, which are responsible for clearing out misfolded and toxic peptides, promote the accumulation of htt fragments in aged neurons. In the meantime, an expanded polyglutamine tract causes them to misfold and aggregate in the nucleus and neuronal processes. The accumulation of mutant htt in the nucleus and neuronal processes therefore suggests that these subcellular regions are the primary sites for mutant htt to elicit its toxicity.

2.4. NUCLEAR EFFECT OF MUTANT HUNTINGTIN

The nuclear inclusions of mutant htt led investigators to study the mechanisms for this phenomenon. Although some immunostaining and nuclear fractionation studies have shown that normal htt is also localized in the nucleus (*Hoogeveen, Willemsen et al., 1993; Kegel, Meloni et al., 2002*), it is clear that the majority remains in the cytoplasm. Moreover, nuclear htt aggregates can only be recognized by antibodies against the N-terminal region of htt (*DiFiglia, Sapp et al., 1997; Gutekunst, Li et al., 1999*). Furthermore, isolation of nuclear fractions from HD knock-in mice, which express full-length mutant htt under the endogenous mouse HD gene, provides evidence that multiple N-terminal htt fragments accumulate in the nucleus (*Zhou, Cao et al., 2003*). The association between nuclear accumulation of mutant htt and disease progression is clear from several HD mouse models. In HD knock-in mouse models, mutant htt accumulates preferentially in the nuclei of striatal neurons and forms more prominent aggregates as disease progresses (*Wheeler, White et al., 2000; Lin, Tallaksen-Greene et al., 2001*). A progressive phenotype is also associated with the nuclear accumulation of an amino-terminal cleavage fragment in a transgenic mouse model with inducible expression of full-length mutant huntingtin (*Tanaka, Igarashi et al., 2006*). Targeting mutant htt with nuclear localization sequences to direct mutant htt in the nucleus of mouse brains produces neurological phenotypes (*Schilling, Savonenko et al., 2004; Benn, Landles et al., 2005*). Moreover, prevention of htt cleavage by mutating caspase-6 site can alleviate neurological phenotypes and delay the nuclear accumulation of mutant htt in AC transgenic mice (*Graham, Deng et al., 2006*).

Studies of N-terminal htt fragments have failed to find that these fragments contain nuclear localizations sequences. Thus, N-terminal htt fragments may passively enter the nucleus, but expanded polyQ repeats prevent their export from the nucleus (*Cornett, Cao et al., 2005*). The presence of mutant htt fragments in the nucleus and various cleavage sites in the N-terminal region of htt (*Sun, Savanenin et al., 2001*) also support the notion that proteolysis of htt leads to the generation of toxic htt fragments. Consistently, smaller N-terminal htt fragments appear to be more toxic than large-sized fragments in both cultured cells (*Hackam, Singaraja et al., 1998*) and transgenic animals (*Davies, Turmaine et al., 1997; Schilling, Becher et al., 1999; Yu, Li et al., 2003*).

The aberrant nuclear accumulation of mutant htt is likely to cause gene transcriptional dysregulations. Indeed, several nuclear transcription factors are found to bind htt (*Sugars and Rubinsztein 2003; Li and Li 2004*). Of these, the coactivators cAMP response element-binding protein (CREB)-binding protein (CBP) and the specificity protein 1 (Sp1) are particularly important for neuronal function. Deletion of CREB in the brain causes selective neurodegeneration in the hippocampus and striatum (*Mantamadiotis, Lemberger et al., 2002*). Many neuronal genes that lack a TATA box require Sp1 for their transcription (*Myers, Dingledine et al., 1999*). Dysregulation of gene expression mediated by CBP and Sp1 have been found in HD mouse brains (*Luthi-Carter, Hanson et al., 2002*).

The interactions of mutant htt with transcription factors may occur at various binding sites. Many transcription factors contain a polyQ-rich domain. Since CBP is recruited into aggregates formed by different polyQ proteins, such as the androgen receptor (*McCampbell, Taylor et al., 2000*), the SCA3

(*Chai, Wu et al., 2001*), and the Dentatorubral-Pallidoluysian atrophy (DRPLA) proteins (*Nucifora, Sasaki et al., 2001*), it has been thought that the polyQ domain is the binding site to interact with other polyQ proteins. Supporting this idea, a number of transcription factors containing polyQ or proline –rich domains, including CBP (*Nucifora, Sasaki et al., 2001; Steffan, Bodai et al., 2001*), TBP (*Huang, Faber et al., 1998; Perez, Paulson et al., 1998*), and TAF130 (*Shimohata, Nakajima et al., 2000*), have been found in nuclear polyQ inclusions.

However, subsequent studies showed that the acetyltransferase domain in CBP interacts with htt (*Chai, Wu et al., 2001; Steffan, Bodai et al., 2001*), which led to the finding that inhibition of histone deacetylase (HDAC) or promotion of histone acetylation ameliorates neurodegeneration in cellular and fly models (*Steffan, Bodai et al., 2001*) and motor deficits in a mouse model of HD (*Hockly, Richon et al., 2003*).

These observations prompted a hypothesis whereby the pathogenic process was linked to the state of histone acetylation; specifically, mutant huntingtin induced a state of reduced histone acetylation and as a result altered gene expression. Support for this idea was obtained from the Drosophila HD model expressing an N-terminal fragment of huntingtin with an expanded polyglutamine tract in the eye. Administration of inhibitors of histone deacetylation (HDAC) arrested neurodegeneration and lethality (*Steffan, Bodai et al., 2001*). Hughes et al. in 2002 reported protective effects of HDAC inhibitors for other polyglutamine disorders, prompting the concept that at least some of the observed effects in polyglutamine-disorders are due to alterations in histone acetylation. This hypothesis has led to several preclinical studies using HDAC inhibitors (*Ferrante and Kubilus 2003, Gardian, Browne et al., 2005*).

Whether HDAC inhibitors, such as the FDA-approved SAHA, can be used in treating HD and other polyglutamine disorders remains to be seen. The evidence linking histone acetylation to polyglutamine pathogenesis is based for the most part on work performed using a fragment of the mutant polyglutamine protein. Thus, the biological relevance of this work depends on the extent to which the pathogenesis will prove to rest on the properties of the polyglutamine tract.

The colocalization of some transcription factors in nuclear polyQ inclusions also led to the idea that recruitment of transcription factors into polyQ inclusions reduces the level of these transcription factors. However, after examining several HD mouse models, researchers were unable to find decreased levels of CBP in symptomatic mouse brains (*Yu, Li et al., 2002;*

Tallaksen-Greene, Crouse et al., 2005). In addition altered expression of a number of genes was not necessarily associated with the formation of htt aggregates in HD mice (*Luthi-Carter, Hanson et al., 2002*) and were apt to occur in cell models in the absence of nuclear inclusions (*Kita, Carmichael et al., 2002; Sipione, Rigamonti et al., 2002*). Thus, it is likely that soluble or misfolded htt may interact with transcription factors to alter transcriptional activity. This idea is further supported by the finding that soluble mutant htt reduces the binding of Sp1 to DNA (*Dunah, Jeong et al., 2002; Li, Cheng et al., 2002*).

Combined, there is ample evidence that mutant htt acts in the nucleus to affect gene transcription (**Transcriptional dysregulation hypothesis**)

2.5. Cytoplasmic Effect of Mutant Huntingtin

A. Axonal Transport in HD

Earlier studies have reported that mutant htt not only increases caspase activity (*Ona, Li et al., 1999; Sanchez, Xu et al., 1999; Chen, Ona et al., 2000; Li, Lam et al., 2000*) but also affects various signaling pathways (*Cepeda, Ariano et al., 2001; Song, Perides et al., 2002; Zeron, Hansson et al., 2002; Tang, Tu et al., 2003*). These findings suggest that mutant htt also acts in the cytoplasm to affect cellular functions (Figure 8: Molecular and cellular pathways involved in HD pathogenesis).

Therefore, an intensive search to reveal the interactions between htt and cytoplasm proteins began. By means of the yeast two-hybrid screen and in vivo binding assays, a number of cytoplasmic proteins were found to interact with htt (*Sharp, Loev et al., 1995; Harjes and Wanker 2003; Borrell-Pages, Zala et al., 2006*). Of these, htt associated protein 1 (HAP1) and htt-interacting protein 1 (HIP1) have been studied extensively. Both proteins may well be involved in intracellular trafficking. HAP1 binds more tightly to mutant htt than to normal htt (*Li, Li et al., 1995*) HAP1 also associates with both dynactin p150, which is involved in microtubule-dependent retrograde transport (*Engelender, Sharp et al., 1997; Li, Gutekunst et al., 1998*), and kinesin light chain 2 (*McGuire, Rong et al., 2006*), which is involved in anterograde transport. Several studies suggest that HAP1 participates in the trafficking or endocytosis of membrane receptors, including those for epidermal growth factor (*Li, Chin et al., 2002*), type 1 inositol (1,4,5) –triphosphate receptor (InsP3R1) (*Tang, Tu et al., 2003*), GABA (*Kittler, Thomas et al., 2004*),and nerve growth factor (NGF) (*Rong, McGuire et al., 2006*). Like htt, HAP1 is located at various subcellular sites, including microtubules and synaptic vesicles in axonal terminals (*Gutekunst, Li et al., 1998*). Mice lacking HAP1 often die at postnatal day 3 (*Chan, Nasir et al., 2002; Li, Yu et al., 2003*), which is likely due to neuronal degeneration in the hypothalamus (*Li, Yu et al., 2003*). The hypothalamic function of HAP1 appears to be critical for feeding behavior and metabolism (*Sheng, Chang et al., 2006*), and its dysfunction may contribute to hypothalamic pathology or degeneration in HD (*Kremer, Roos et al., 1990; Li, Yu et al., 2003; Petersen, Gil et al., 2005; Sheng, Chang et al., 2006*).

HIP1 is also important for assembly and function of the cytoskeleton and endocytosis (*Kalchman, Koide et al., 1997*) and binds clathrin and alpha-adaptin subunit AP-2 (*Mishra, Agostinelli et al., 2001; Waelter, Scherzinger et al., 2001; Metzler, Li et al., 2003*). The interactions of HIP1 with these proteins may constitute a protein complex involved in clathrin-mediated endocytosis. Unlike HAP1, HIP1 binds mutant htt weakly (*Kalchman, Koide et al., 1997*). This finding suggests that HIP1 requires interaction with htt for normal function, whereas dissociation from mutant htt may impair its function.

Although the interactions of htt with HAP1, HIP1, and other cytoplasmic proteins suggests that htt is involved in intracellular trafficking, more compelling evidence has come from the studies of trafficking function in cells that express mutant htt. Recent studies show that normal Drosophila htt functions in the axonal transport pathway and that polyQ expansion causes soluble htt to recruit more microtubule transporter proteins, thereby reducing the soluble pool of these proteins in axons (*Gunawardena, Her et al., 2003*). In cultured neurons, htt is involved in HAP1-associated axonal transport of brain-derived neurotrophic factor (BDNF), both anterogradely and retrogradely, which is disrupted by mutant htt (*Gauthier, Charrin et al., 2004*).

The presence of an expanded polyglutamine tract in huntingtin increases the interaction between huntingtin, HAP1, and p150 Glued and thereby reduces the interaction of HAP1/p150 Glued with microtubules, which most likely accounts for the decrease in transport in the presence of mutant huntingtin. This mutant huntingtin-induced reduction in BDNF-containing vesicle transport reduces trophic support, causing neurotoxicity, which may contribute to the pathogenesis of HD. Recent studies (*Colin, Zala et al., 2008*) have demonstrated that Huntingtin is a positive regulatory factor for vesicular transport. Huntingtin is phosphorylated at serine 421 by the kinase Akt, and this event seems to be crucial to control the direction of vesicles in neurons. When phosphorylated, huntingtin recruits kinesin-1 to the dynactin complex on vesicles and microtubules promoting anterograde transport. Conversely, when huntingtin is not phosphorylated, kinesin-1 detaches and vesicles are more likely to undergo retrograde transport. This also applies to other vesicles suggesting an essential role for huntingtin in the control of vesicular directionality in neurons.

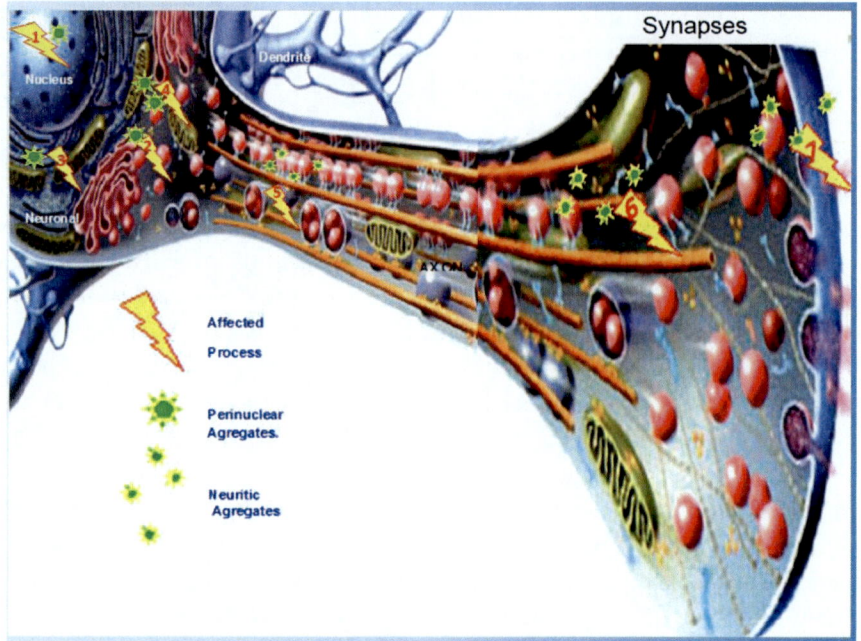

A hypothetical model of proposed molecular and cellular mechanisms involved in the pathogenesis of HD. The expanded polyglutamine in the mutant HD protein is proposed to disrupt key processes relating to cell signaling (4), gene transcription (1), protein trafficking (2, 5, 6), presynaptic and postsynaptic signaling (7), mitochondrial dysfunction (3) and protein-protein interactions.

Figure 8. Molecular and cellular pathways involved in HD pathogenesis.

Moreover, there are multiple evidences which confirm that phosphorylation of htt at serine 421 (S421) restores its function in axonal transport. Using a strategy involving RNA (ribonucleic acid) interference and re-expression of various constructs, Zala, Colin et al. (2008) demonstrated that polyQ (polyglutamine)-htt is unable to promote transport of brain-derived neurotrophic factor (BDNF)-containing vesicles, but polyQ-htt constitutively phosphorylated at S421 is as effective as the wild-type (wt) as concerns transport of these vesicles. The S421 phosphorylated polyQ-htt displays the wt function of inducing BDNF release. Phosphorylation restores the interaction between htt and the p150(Glued) subunit of dynactin and their association with microtubules in vitro and in cells. This is the first description of a mechanism that restores the htt function altered in disease.

B. Mitochondrial/Bioenergetic Dysfunction and HD

Investigators have long thought that mitochondrial dysfunction plays an important role in neurodegenerative diseases. The strongest evidence that a mutant polyglutamine protein may have a direct effect on mitochondrial function is for HD. That mitochondrial defects may be a direct effect of mutant huntingtin stems from studies demonstrating mitochondrial Ca+ defects in HD material (*Tang, Slow, et al. 2005*). Panov et al. found (2002) that mitochondria isolated from lymphoblasts of HD patients and mitochondria isolated from the brains of mice expressing full-length mutant huntingtin had a similar deficit in membrane potential and depolarization in response to Ca+ loading. In the mice this deficit preceded onset of disease, and they found an N-terminal fragment of huntingtin at the mitochondrial membrane. Incubation of normal mitochondria with this N-terminal mutant huntingtin fragment induces the mitochondrial defects seen in HD patients and transgenic mice. In addition to altering calcium signaling at the mitochondrial membrane, Tang et al found that mutant huntingtin affects Ca+ signaling, leading to cytoplasmic Ca+ overload by sensitizing the InsP3R1 to activation by InsP3. Enhanced release of proapoptotic factors such as cytochrome C from mitochondria in medium spiny neurons was speculated to lead to apoptosis and HD.

A potentially important finding is the recent report of a relationship between the polyglutamine tract length and the cellular energy status (*Seong, Ivanova, et al. 2005*). In this study the investigators first examined the ATP levels in a striatal cell line generated from mice carrying an expanded CAG inserted into the endogenous mouse SCA 1 gene and found low mitochondrial ATP production and a decrease in the ability of the mitochondria to take up ADP. An analysis of the ATP/ADP ratio in 40 human lymphoblast cell lines generated from individuals with CAG repeats spanning a size from normal (9-34 repeats) to affected (35-70 repeats) alleles revealed an inverse association between the length of the longest repeat in an individual and the ATP/ADP ratio. This association extended throughout both the normal and mutant alleles, indicating that the length of the polyglutamine tract in huntingtin, in some fashion, regulates the energy status of a cell that may contribute to the increased susceptibility of striatal neurons in HD.

Recent studies (*Lee, Ivanova, et al. 2007*) were performed to test the prevailing hypothesis that huntingtin may directly affect the mitochondrion. By using comprehensive gene expression analysis, it was investigated whether the HD mutation may replicate the effects of 3-nitropropionic acid (3-NP), a compound known to inhibit mitochondria, with loss of striatal neurons. They found that, while mutant huntingtin and 3-NP both elicited energy starvation, the gene responses to the HD mutation, unlike the responses to 3-NP, did not highlight damage to mitochondria, but instead revealed effects on huntingtin-dependent processes. Thus, rather than direct inhibition, the polyglutamine tract size appears to modulate some normal activity of huntingtin that indirectly influences the management of the mitochondrion. Understanding the precise nature of this extra-mitochondrial process would critically guide efforts to achieve effective energy-based therapeutics in HD.

Chapter 3

CONCLUSION

Huntington's disease appears to involve disruption of numerous molecular and cellular processes, including protein-protein interactions, proteosomal actions, transcriptional regulation, protein trafficking, inter and intraneuronal signaling and synaptic plasticity. This disruption is expressed as an altered structure and function of networks of neurons, leading to motor, cognitive and psychiatric symptoms, prior to overt cell death. The role of other specific cellular processes, such as altered neurogenesis, may either be an epiphenomenon or a causative component of pathogenesis and this remains one of the many issues yet to be fully elucidated. A key issue for further investigation is to distinguish cause and effect with respect to mechanisms of pathogenesis.

Other important issue facing researchers is how to sort out the major pathogenic pathways as targets for developing therapeutic strategies. For example, which is the more critical for neuronal dysfunction and neurodegeneration, the nuclear or cytoplasmic effect of mutant htt?

Answering this question would require a better understanding than we currently possess of mutant htt's effects in different type of cells and at different stages of disease.

Identification of molecular pathways altered by expanded repeats is beginning to reveal potential therapeutic interventions that can be tested in the existing animal models in preparation for eventual clinical investigations. The findings that motor, behavioral, and pathological phenotypes can be reversed in mouse models of HD upon silencing of the mutant transgene are quite exciting and provide hope that therapeutic interventions will likely benefit not only presymptomatic individuals, but potentially individuals in early and midstages of the disease as well.

REFERENCES

Al-Jader, L. N. & Harper, P. S. et al. (2001). "The frequency of inherited disorders database: prevalence of Huntington disease." *Community Genet. 4(3)*, 148-57.

Andrade, M. A. & Bork, P. (1995). "HEAT repeats in the Huntington´s disease protein". *Nat. Genet. 11*, 115-116.

Andrew, S. E. & Goldberg, Y. P. et al. (1993). "The relationship between trinucleotide (CAG) repeat length and clinical features of Huntington's disease." *Nat. Genet. 4(4)*, 398-403.

Arrasate, M. & Mitra, S. et al. (2004). "Inclusion body formation reduces levels of mutant huntingtin and the risk of neuronal death." *Nature. 431(7010)*, 805-10.

Benn, C. L. & Landles C. et al. (2005). "Contribution of nuclear and extranuclear polyQ to neurological phenotypes in mouse models of Huntington's disease." *Hum. Mol. Genet. 14(20)*, 3065-78.

Bertram, L. & Tanzi, R. E. (2005). "The genetic epidemiology of neurodegenerative disease." *J. Clin. Invest. 115(6)*, 1449-57.

Bodner, R. A. & Housman, D. E. et al. (2006). "New directions for neurodegenerative disease therapy: using chemical compounds to boost the formation of mutant protein inclusions." *Cell Cycle. 5(14)*, 1477-80.

Bodner, R. A. & Outeiro, T. F. et al. (2006). "Pharmacological promotion of inclusion formation: a therapeutic approach for Huntington's and Parkinson's diseases." *Proc. Natl. Acad. Sci. U. S. A. 103(11)*, 4246-51.

Borrell-Pages, M. & Zala D. et al. (2006). "Huntington's disease: from huntingtin function and dysfunction to therapeutic strategies." *Cell. Mol. Life Sci. 63(22)*, 2642-60.

Brais, B., Bouchard, J. P., Xie, Y. G., Rochefort, D. L. & Chretien, N. et al. (1998). "Short GCG expansions in the PABP2 gene cause oculopharyngeal muscular dystrophy." *Nat. Genet.* 18, 164-67. Erratum, 1998. *Nat. Genet., 19 (4),* 404.

Brinkman, R. R. & Mezei, M. M. et al. (1997). "The likelihood of being affected with Huntington disease by a particular age, for a specific CAG size." *Am. J. Hum. Genet. 60(5),* 1202-10.

Butler, R. and G. P. Bates (2006). "Histone deacetylase inhibitors as therapeutics for polyglutamine disorders." *Nat. Rev. Neurosci. 7(10),* 784-96.

Cattaneo, E., D. Rigamonti, et al. (2001). "Loss of normal huntingtin function: new developments in Huntington's disease research." *Trends Neurosci. 24(3),* 182-8.

Cepeda, C., Ariano M. A., et al. (2001). "NMDA receptor function in mouse models of Huntington disease." *J. Neurosci. Res. 66(4),* 525-39.

Chai, Y., Wu L., et al. (2001). "The role of protein composition in specifying nuclear inclusion formation in polyglutamine disease." *J. Biol. Chem. 276(48),* 44889-97.

Chan, E. Y., Nasir J., et al. (2002). "Targeted disruption of Huntingtin-associated protein-1 (Hap1) results in postnatal death due to depressed feeding behavior." *Hum. Mol. Genet. 11(8),* 945-59.

Chen, M. & Ona V. O. et al. (2000). "Minocycline inhibits caspase-1 and caspase-3 expression and delays mortality in a transgenic mouse model of Huntington disease." *Nat. Med. 6(7),* 797-801.

Colin, E., Zala, D. & Liot, G. et al., (2008). "Huntingtin phosphorylation acts as a molecular switch for anterograde/retrograde transport in neurons". *EMBO J. , 6,* 27(15),2124-34.

Conneally, P. M. & Haines, J. L. et al., (1989). "Huntington disease: no evidence for locus heterogeneity." *Genomics, 5(2),* 304-8.

Cornett, J. & Cao F. et al., (2005). "Polyglutamine expansion of huntingtin impairs its nuclear export." *Nat. Genet. 37(2),* 198-204.

Davies, S. W. & Turmaine, M. et al., (1997). "Formation of neuronal intranuclear inclusions underlies the neurological dysfunction in mice transgenic for the HD mutation." *Cell. 90 (3),* 537-48.

DiFiglia, M. & Sapp E. et al., (1995). "Huntingtin is a cytoplasmic protein associated with vesicles in human and rat brain neurons." *Neuron. 14(5),* 1075-81.

Dragatsis, I. & Levine M. S. et al. (2000). "Inactivation of Hdh in the brain and testis results in progressive neurodegeneration and sterility in mice." *Nat. Genet. 26(3)*, 300-6.

Duff, K. & Beglinger, L. J. et al., (2009). *"Cognitive deficits in Huntington's disease on the Repeatable Battery for the Assessment of Neuropsychological Status". J. Clin. Exp. Neuropsychol. 29,1-9*

Dunah, A. W. & Jeong, H. et al. (2002). "Sp1 and TAFII130 transcriptional activity disrupted in early Huntington's disease." *Science. 296(5576)*, 2238-43.

Duyao, M. P. & Auerbach A. B. et al. (1995). "Inactivation of the mouse Huntington's disease gene homolog Hdh." *Science. 269(5222)*, 407-10.

Engelender, S. & Sharp, A. H. et al. (1997) "Huntingtin-associated protein 1 (HAP1) interacts with the p150Glued subunit of dynactin". *Hum. Mol. Genet.* 6(13), 2205-2212.

Ferrante, R. J. & Kowall N. W. et al., (1985). "Selective sparing of a class of striatal neurons in Huntington's disease." *Science. 230(4725)*, 561-3.

Ferrante, R. J. & Kubilus, J. K. et al. (2003). "Histone deacetylase inhibition by sodium butyrate chemotherapy ameliorates the neurodegeneration phenotype in Huntington's disease mice". *J. Neurosci.*, 23, 9418-27.

Gafni, J. & Ellerby, L. M. (2002). "Calpain activation in Huntington's disease." *J. Neurosci. 22(12)*, 4842-9.

Gardian, G. & Browne, S. E. et al. (2005). "Neuroprotective effects of phenylbutyrate in the N171-82Q trangenic mouse model of Huntington's disease." *J. Biol. Chem.*, 280, 556-63.

Gatchel, J. R. & Zoghbi, H. Y. (2005). "Diseases of unstable repeat expansion: mechanisms and common principles." *Nat. Rev. Genet. 6(10)*, 743-55.

Gauthier, L. R. & Charrin B. C. et al. (2004). "Huntingtin controls neurotrophic support and survival of neurons by enhancing BDNF vesicular transport along microtubules." *Cell. 118(1)*, 127-38.

Graham, R. K. & Deng Y. et al., (2006). "Cleavage at the caspase-6 site is required for neuronal dysfunction and degeneration due to mutant huntingtin." *Cell. 125(6)*, 1179-91.

Graveland, G. A. & Williams R. S. et al., (1985). "Evidence for degenerative and regenerative changes in neostriatal spiny neurons in Huntington's disease." *Science. 227(4688)*, 770-3.

Gu, X. & Li, C. et al., (2005). "Pathological cell-cell interactions elicited by a neuropathogenic form of mutant Huntingtin contribute to cortical pathogenesis in HD mice." *Neuron. 46(3)*, 433-44.

Gunawardena, S. & Her L. S. et al. (2003). "Disruption of axonal transport by loss of huntingtin or expression of pathogenic polyQ proteins in Drosophila." *Neuron. 40(1)*, 25-40.

Gusella, J. F. & Wexler N. S. et al. (1983). "A polymorphic DNA marker genetically linked to Huntington's disease." *Nature. 306(5940)*, 234-8.

Gutekunst, C. A. & Li, S. H. et al. (1999). "Nuclear and neuropil aggregates in Huntington's disease: relationship to neuropathology." *J. Neurosci. 19(7)*, 2522-34.

Gutekunst, C. A. & Norflus F. et al. (2000). "Recent advances in Huntington's disease." *Curr. Opin. Neurol. 13(4)*, 445-50.

Gutekunst, C. A. & Levey A. I. et al. (1995). "Identification and localization of huntingtin in brain and human lymphoblastoid cell lines with anti-fusion protein antibodies." *Proc. Natl. Acad. Sci. U. S. A. 92(19)*, 8710-4.

Gutekunst, C. A. & Li S. H. et al. (1998). "The cellular and subcellular localization of huntingtin-associated protein 1 (HAP1): comparison with huntingtin in rat and human." *J. Neurosci. 18(19)*, 7674-86.

Hackam, A. S. & Singaraja R. et al. (1998). "The influence of huntingtin protein size on nuclear localization and cellular toxicity." *J. Cell Biol. 141(5)*, 1097-105.

Harjes, P. & Wanker E. E. (2003). "The hunt for huntingtin function: interaction partners tell many different stories." *Trends Biochem. Sci. 28(8)*, 425-33.

Harper, P. S. (1992). "The epidemiology of Huntington's disease." *Hum. Genet. 89(4)*, 365-76.

Heinsen, H. & Rub U. et al., (1999). "Nerve cell loss in the thalamic mediodorsal nucleus in Huntington's disease." *Acta Neuropathol.* (Berl) *97(6)*, 613-22.

Hockly, E. & Richon V. M. et al. (2003). "Suberoylanilide hydroxamic acid, a histone deacetylase inhibitor, ameliorates motor deficits in a mouse model of Huntington's disease." *Proc. Natl. Acad. Sci. U. S. A. 100(4)*, 2041-6.

Hodgson, J. G. & Agopyan, N., et al. (1999). "A YAC mouse model for Huntington's disease with full-length mutant huntingtin, cytoplasmic toxicity, and selective striatal neurodegeneration." *Neuron. 23(1)*, 181-92.

Hodgson, J. G. & Smith D. J. et al. (1996). "Human huntingtin derived from YAC transgenes compensates for loss of murine huntingtin by rescue of the embryonic lethal phenotype." *Hum. Mol. Genet. 5(12)*, 1875-85.

Hoogeveen, A. T. & Willemsen R. et al. (1993). "Characterization and localization of the Huntington disease gene product." *Hum. Mol. Genet. 2(12)*, 2069-73.

Huang, C. C. & Faber P. W. et al. (1998). "Amyloid formation by mutant huntingtin, threshold, progressivity and recruitment of normal polyglutamine proteins." *Somat. Cell Mol. Genet. 24(4)*, 217-33.

Hughes, R. E. (2002). "Polyglutamine Disease: acetyltransferases away". *Curr. Biol., 12*, R 141-43.

Ishiguro, H. & Yamada, K. et al. (2001). "Age-dependent and tissue-specific CAG repeat instability occurs in mouse knock-in for a mutant Huntington's disease gene." *J. Neurosci. Res. 65(4)*, 289-97.

Kalchman, M. A. & Koide H. B. et al., (1997). "HIP1, a human homologue of S. cerevisiae Sla2p, interacts with membrane-associated huntingtin in the brain." *Nat. Genet. 16(1)*, 44-53.

Kegel, K. B. & Meloni A. R. et al., (2002). "Huntingtin is present in the nucleus, interacts with the transcriptional corepressor C-terminal binding protein, and represses transcription." *J. Biol. Chem. 277(9)*, 7466-76.

Kenney C., Powell, S. & Jankovic, J. (2007) "Autopsy-proven Huntington´s disease with 29 trinucleotide repeats". *Mov. Disord. 22*, 127-130.

Kim, Y. J. & Yi Y. et al. (2001). "Caspase 3-cleaved N-terminal fragments of wild-type and mutant huntingtin are present in normal and Huntington's disease brains, associate with membranes, and undergo calpain-dependent proteolysis." *Proc. Natl. Acad. Sci. U. S. A. 98(22)*, 12784-9.

Kita, H. & Carmichael J. et al. (2002). "Modulation of polyglutamine-induced cell death by genes identified by expression profiling." *Hum. Mol. Genet. 11(19)*, 2279-87.

Kittler, J. T. & Thomas, P. et al. (2004). "Huntingtin-associated protein 1 regulates inhibitory synaptic transmission by modulating gamma-aminobutyric acid type A receptor membrane trafficking." *Proc. Natl. Acad. Sci. U. S. A. 101(34)*, 12736-41.

Kremer, B. & Squitieri, F. et al., (1993). "Molecular analysis of late onset Huntington´s disease". *J. Med. Genet., 30*, 991-995.

Kremer, H. P. & Roos R. A. et al., (1990). "Atrophy of the hypothalamic lateral tuberal nucleus in Huntington's disease." *J. Neuropathol. Exp. Neurol. 49(4)*, 371-82.

Kuemmerle, S. & Gutekunst C. A. et al. (1999). "Huntington aggregates may not predict neuronal death in Huntington's disease." *Ann. Neurol. 46(6)*, 842-9.

Lee J. M. & Ivanova E. V. et al., (2007). "Unbiased gene expression analysis implicates the huntingtin polyglutamine tract in extra-mitochondrial energy metabolism." *PLoS Genet., 3(8)*, e135.

Li S. H. & Gutekunst C. A., et al., (1998). " Interaction of huntingtin-associated protein with dynactin P150Glued." *J. Neurosci.* 18, 1261-1269.

Li, H. & Li, S. H. et al. (1999). "Ultrastructural localization and progressive formation of neuropil aggregates in Huntington's disease transgenic mice." *Hum. Mol. Genet. 8(7)*, 1227-36.

Li, H. & Li, S. H. et al. (2000). "Amino-terminal fragments of mutant huntingtin show selective accumulation in striatal neurons and synaptic toxicity." *Nat. Genet. 25(4)*, 385-9.

Li, H. & Li, S. H. et al. (2001). "Huntingtin aggregate-associated axonal degeneration is an early pathological event in Huntington's disease mice." *J. Neurosci. 21(21)*, 8473-81.

Li, S. H. & Li, X. J. (1998). "Aggregation of N-terminal huntingtin is dependent on the length of its glutamine repeats." *Hum. Mol. Genet. 7(5)*, 777-82.

Li, S. H. & Li, X. J. (2004). "Huntingtin-protein interactions and the pathogenesis of Huntington's disease." *Trends Genet. 20(3)*, 146-54.

Li, S. H. & Cheng, A. L. et al. (2002). "Interaction of Huntington disease protein with transcriptional activator Sp1." *Mol. Cell Biol. 22(5)*, 1277-87.

Li, S. H. & Gutekunst, C. A. et al. (1998). "Interaction of huntingtin-associated protein with dynactin P150Glued." *J. Neurosci. 18(4)*, 1261-9.

Li, S. H. & Lam S. et al. (2000). "Intranuclear huntingtin increases the expression of caspase-1 and induces apoptosis." *Hum. Mol. Genet. 9(19)*, 2859-67.

Li, S. H. & Yu, Z. X. et al. (2003). "Lack of huntingtin-associated protein-1 causes neuronal death resembling hypothalamic degeneration in Huntington's disease." *J. Neurosci. 23(17)*, 6956-64.

Li, X. J. & Li, S. H. et al. (1995). "A huntingtin-associated protein enriched in brain with implications for pathology." *Nature. 378(6555)*, 398-402.

Li, Y. & Chin, L. S. et al. (2002). "Huntingtin-associated protein 1 interacts with hepatocyte growth factor-regulated tyrosine kinase substrate and functions in endosomal trafficking." *J. Biol. Chem. 277(31)*, 28212-21.

Lin, C. H. & Tallaksen-Greene, S. et al. (2001). "Neurological abnormalities in a knock-in mouse model of Huntington's disease." *Hum. Mol. Genet. 10(2)*, 137-44.

Lipe H. & Bird, T. (2009). "Late onset Huntington Disease: clinical and genetic characteristics of 34 cases". *J. Neurol. Sci., 276(1-2),159-62.*

Lodi, R. & Schapira, A. H. et al., (2000). "Abnormal in vivo skeletal muscle energy metabolism in Huntington´s disease and dentatorubropallidoluysian atrophy". *Ann. Neurol. 48*,72-76.

Lunkes, A. & Lindenberg, K. S. et al. (2002). "Proteases acting on mutant huntingtin generate cleaved products that differentially build up cytoplasmic and nuclear inclusions." *Mol. Cell. 10(2)*, 259-69.

Luthi-Carter, R. & Hanson, S. A. et al. (2002). "Dysregulation of gene expression in the R6/2 model of polyglutamine disease: parallel changes in muscle and brain." *Hum. Mol. Genet. 11(17)*, 1911-26.

MacDonald, M. E. & Novelletto, A. et al. (1992). "The Huntington's disease candidate region exhibits many different haplotypes." *Nat. Genet. 1(2)*, 99-103.

MacDonald, V. & Halliday, G. (2002). "Pyramidal cell loss in motor cortices in Huntington's disease." *Neurobiol Dis, 10(3)*, 378-86.

Mantamadiotis, T. & Lemberger, T. et al. (2002). "Disruption of CREB function in brain leads to neurodegeneration." *Nat Genet, 31(1)*, 47-54.

Marder, K. & Zhao, H. et al., (2009). "Dietary intake in adults at risk for Huntington disease: analysis of PHAROS research participants". *Neurology. 73(5)*, 385-92.

McCampbell, A. & Taylor, J. P. et al. (2000). "CREB-binding protein sequestration by expanded polyglutamine." *Hum. Mol. Genet. 9(14)*, 2197-202.

McGuire, J. R. & Rong J. et al. (2006). "Interaction of Huntingtin-associated protein-1 with kinesin light chain: implications in intracellular trafficking in neurons." *J. Biol. Chem. 281(6)*, 3552-9.

McNeil, S. M. & Novelletto, A. et al. (1997). "Reduced penetrance of the Huntington's disease mutation." *Hum. Mol. Genet. 6(5)*, 775-9.

Menalled, L. B. & Sison J. D. et al. (2003). "Time course of early motor and neuropathological anomalies in a knock-in mouse model of Huntington's disease with 140 CAG repeats." *J. Comp. Neurol. 465(1)*, 11-26.

Menalled, L. B. & Sison J. D. et al. (2002). "Early motor dysfunction and striosomal distribution of huntingtin microaggregates in Huntington's disease knock-in mice." *J. Neurosci. 22(18)*, 8266-76.

Metzler, M. & Li, B. et al. (2003). "Disruption of the endocytic protein HIP1 results in neurological deficits and decreased AMPA receptor trafficking." *Embo J. 22(13)*, 3254-66.

Mishra, S. K. & Agostinelli, N. R. et al. (2001). "Clathrin- and AP-2-binding sites in HIP1 uncover a general assembly role for endocytic accessory proteins." *J. Biol. Chem. 276(49)*, 46230-6.

Myers, R. H. & Leavitt, J. et al. (1989). "Homozygote for Huntington disease." *Am. J. Hum. Genet. 45(4)*, 615-8.

Myers, R. H. & MacDonald, M. E. et al. (1993). "De novo expansion of a (CAG)n repeat in sporadic Huntington's disease." *Nat. Genet. 5(2)*, 168-73.

Myers, R. H. & Sax, D. S. et al. (1985). "Late onset of Huntington's disease." *J. Neurol. Neurosurg. Psychiatry. 48(6)*, 530-4.

Myers, R. H. & Sax D. S. et al. (1991). "Factors associated with slow progression in Huntington's disease." *Arch. Neurol. 48(8)*, 800-4.

Myers, R. H. & Vonsattel, J. P. et al. (1991). "Decreased neuronal and increased oligodendroglial densities in Huntington's disease caudate nucleus." *J. Neuropathol. Exp. Neurol. 50(6)*, 729-42.

Myers, S. J. & Dingledine, R., et al. (1999). "Genetic regulation of glutamate receptor ion channels." *Annu. Rev. Pharmacol. Toxicol. 39*, 221-41.

Nasir, J. & Floresco, S. B. et al. (1995). "Targeted disruption of the Huntington's disease gene results in embryonic lethality and behavioral and morphological changes in heterozygotes." *Cell. 81(5)*, 811-23.

Neuwald, A. F. & Hirano, T. (2000). "HEAT repeats associated with condensins, cohesins, and other complexes involved in chromosome-related functions." *Genome Res. 10(10)*, 1445-52.

Nucifora, F. C. & Jr., Sasaki, M. et al. (2001). "Interference by huntingtin and atrophin-1 with cbp-mediated transcription leading to cellular toxicity." *Science. 291(5512)*, 2423-8.

Ona, V. O. & Li, M. et al., (1999). "Inhibition of caspase-1 slows disease progression in a mouse model of Huntington's disease." *Nature. 399(6733)*, 263-7.

Panov A. V. & Gutekunst, C. A. et al., (2002) "Early mitochondrial calcium defects in Huntington's disease are a direct effect of polyglutamines". *Nat. Neurosci., 5(8)*,731-6.

Peinemann, A. & Schuller, S. et al., (2005). "Executive dysfunction in early stages of Huntington's disease is associated with striatal and insular atrophy, A neuropsychological and voxel-based morphometric study". *J. Neurol. Sci., 239(1),11-9*.

Perez, M. K. & Paulson, H. L. et al. (1998). "Recruitment and the role of nuclear localization in polyglutamine-mediated aggregation." *J. Cell Biol. 143(6)*, 1457-70.

Petersen, A. & Gil, J. et al. (2005). "Orexin loss in Huntington's disease." *Hum. Mol. Genet. 14(1)*, 39-47.

Rajkowska, G. & Selemon, L. D. et al. (1998). "Neuronal and glial somal size in the prefrontal cortex: a postmortem morphometric study of schizophrenia and Huntington disease." *Arch. Gen. Psychiatry. 55(3)*, 215-24.

Ranen N. G. & Stine C. O. et al. (1995). "Anticipation and instability of IT-15 (CAG)n repeats in parent-offspring pairs with Huntington's disease. *Am. J. Hum. Genet.*, *57*, 593-602.

Reddy, P. H. & Williams, M. et al. (1998). "Behavioural abnormalities and selective neuronal loss in HD transgenic mice expressing mutated full-length HD cDNA." *Nat. Genet. 20(2)*, 198-202.

Rong, J. & McGuire, J. R. et al., (2006). "Regulation of intracellular trafficking of huntingtin-associated protein-1 is critical for TrkA protein levels and neurite outgrowth." *J. Neurosci. 26(22)*, 6019-30.

Rosas H. D. & Koroshetz, W. J. et al. (2003). "Evidence for more widespread cerebral pathology in early HD: An MRI-based morphometric analysis". *Neurology. 60*, 1615-20.

Rosenblatt, A. & Abbott, M. H. et al., (2003). "Predictors of neuropathological severity in 100 patients with Huntington´s disease". *Ann. Neurol.*, *54*, 488-93.

Rubinsztein, D. C. & Barton, D. E. et al. (1993). "Analysis of the huntingtin gene reveals a trinucleotide-length polymorphism in the region of the gene that contains two CCG-rich stretches and a correlation between decreased age of onset of Huntington's disease and CAG repeat number." *Hum. Mol. Genet. 2(10)*, 1713-5.

Sanchez, I. & Xu, C. J. et al. (1999). "Caspase-8 is required for cell death induced by expanded polyglutamine repeats." *Neuron. 22(3)*, 623-33.

Sapp, E. & Kegel, K. B. et al. (2001). "Early and progressive accumulation of reactive microglia in the Huntington disease brain." *J. Neuropathol. Exp. Neurol. 60(2)*, 161-72.

Saudou, F. & Finkbeiner, S. et al. (1998). "Huntingtin acts in the nucleus to induce apoptosis but death does not correlate with the formation of intranuclear inclusions." *Cell. 95(1)*, 55-66.

Schilling, G. & Becher, M. W. et al. (1999). "Intranuclear inclusions and neuritic aggregates in transgenic mice expressing a mutant N-terminal fragment of huntingtin." *Hum. Mol. Genet. 8(3)*, 397-407.

Schilling, G. & Savonenko, A. V. et al. (2004). "Nuclear-targeting of mutant huntingtin fragments produces Huntington's disease-like phenotypes in transgenic mice." *Hum. Mol. Genet. 13(15)*, 1599-610.

Semaka, A. & Creighton, S. et al., (2006) "Predictive testing for Huntington disease: interpretation and significance of intermediate alleles". *Clin. Genet.*, *70*, 283-94.

Seong, I. S. & Ivanova, E. et al. (2005)."HD CAG repeat implicates a dominant property of huntingtin in mitochondrial energy metabolism". *Hum. Mol. Genet., 14(19),2871-80.*

Sharp, A. H., Loev, S. J., et al. (1995). "Widespread expression of Huntington's disease gene (IT15) protein product." *Neuron. 14(5),* 1065-74.

Shelbourne, P. F. & Killeen, N. et al. (1999). "A Huntington's disease CAG expansion at the murine Hdh locus is unstable and associated with behavioural abnormalities in mice." *Hum. Mol. Genet. 8(5),* 763-74.

Sheng, G. & Chang, G. Q. et al. (2006). "Hypothalamic huntingtin-associated protein 1 as a mediator of feeding behavior." *Nat. Med. 12(5),* 526-33.

Shimohata, T. & Nakajima, T. et al. (2000). "Expanded polyglutamine stretches interact with TAFII130, interfering with CREB-dependent transcription." *Nat. Genet. 26(1),* 29-36.

Singhrao, S. K. & Thomas, P. et al. (1998). "Huntingtin protein colocalizes with lesions of neurodegenerative diseases: An investigation in Huntington's, Alzheimer's, and Pick's diseases." *Exp. Neurol. 150(2),* 213-22.

Sipione, S. & Rigamonti, D. et al. (2002). "Early transcriptional profiles in huntingtin-inducible striatal cells by microarray analyses." *Hum. Mol. Genet. 11(17),* 1953-65.

Slow, E. J. & Graham, R. K., et al. (2005). "Absence of behavioral abnormalities and neurodegeneration in vivo despite widespread neuronal huntingtin inclusions." *Proc. Natl. Acad. Sci. U. S. A. 102(32),* 11402-7.

Song, C. & Perides, G. et al. (2002). "Expression of full-length polyglutamine-expanded Huntingtin disrupts growth factor receptor signaling in rat pheochromocytoma (PC12) cells." *J. Biol. Chem. 277(8),* 6703-7.

Steffan, J. S. & Bodai, L. et al. (2001). "Histone deacetylase inhibitors arrest polyglutamine-dependent neurodegeneration in Drosophila." *Nature. 413(6857),* 739-43.

Strand, A. D., Aragaki, A. K., Shaw, D., Bird, T., Holton, J. & Turner, C. et al. (2005). "Gene expression in Huntington´s disease skeletal muscle: a potential biomarker". *Hum. Mol. Genet.* 14,1863- 1876.

Stromme, P. & Mangelsdorf, M. E. et al,. (2002). "Mutations in the human ortholog of the Aristaless cause X-linked mental retardation and epilepsy. *Nat. Genet., 30,* 441-45.

Sudarsky, L., Myers, R. H. & Walshe, T. M. (1983). "Huntington´s disease in monozygotic twins reared apart". *J. Med. Genet., 20,* 408-411.

References

Sugars, K. L. & Rubinsztein, D. C. (2003). "Transcriptional abnormalities in Huntington disease." *Trends Genet, 19(5)*, 233-8.

Sun, Y. & Savanenin, A. et al. (2001). "Polyglutamine-expanded huntingtin promotes sensitization of N-methyl-D-aspartate receptors via post-synaptic density 95." *J. Biol. Chem. 276(27)*, 24713-8.

Takano, H. & Gusella, J. F. (2002). "The predominantly HEAT-like motif structure of huntingtin and its association and coincident nuclear entry with dorsal, an NF-kB/Rel/dorsal family transcription factor." *BMC Neurosci. 3*, 15.

Tallaksen-Greene, S. J. & Crouse, A. B. et al. (2005). "Neuronal intranuclear inclusions and neuropil aggregates in HdhCAG(150) knockin mice." *Neuroscience, 131(4)*, 843-52.

Tanaka, Y. & Igarashi, S. et al. (2006). "Progressive phenotype and nuclear accumulation of an amino-terminal cleavage fragment in a transgenic mouse model with inducible expression of full-length mutant huntingtin." *Neurobiol. Dis. 21(2)*, 381-91.

Tang T. S. & Slow, E. et al., (2005). "Disturbed Ca2+ signaling and apoptosis of medium spiny neurons in Huntington's disease". *Proc. Natl. Acad. Sci. U. S. A. 102(7)*, 2602-7.

Tang, T. S. & Tu, H. et al. (2003). "Huntingtin and huntingtin-associated protein 1 influence neuronal calcium signaling mediated by inositol-(1,4,5) triphosphate receptor type 1." *Neuron. 39(2)*, 227-39.

The Huntington's Disease Collaborative Research Group (1993). "A novel gene containing a trinucleotide repeat that is expanded and unstable on Huntington's disease chromosomes". *Cell. 72*, 971-983.

Turner, C. & Cooper, J. M. et al., (2007). "Clinical correlates of mitochondrial function in Huntington´s disease muscle". *Mov. Disord. 22(12)*, 1715-21.

Utsch, B. & Becker, K. et al., (2002)." A novel stable polyalanine (poly A) expansion in the HOXA 13 gene associated with hand-foot-genital syndrome: Proper function of poly (A)-harbouring transcription factors depends on a critical repeat length?". *Hum. Genet., 110*, 488-94.

Vonsattel, J. P. & DiFiglia, M. (1998). "Huntington disease." *J. Neuropathol. Exp. Neurol. 57(5),* 369-84.

Vonsattel, J. P. & Myers, R. H. et al. (1985). "Neuropathological classification of Huntington's disease." *J. Neuropathol. Exp. Neurol. 44(6)*, 559-77.

Waelter, S. & Scherzinger, E. et al. (2001). "The huntingtin interacting protein HIP1 is a clathrin and alpha-adaptin-binding protein involved in receptor-mediated endocytosis." *Hum. Mol. Genet. 10(17)*, 1807-17.

Wellington, C. L. & Ellerby, L. M. et al. (2002). "Caspase cleavage of mutant huntingtin precedes neurodegeneration in Huntington's disease." *J. Neurosci. 22(18)*, 7862-72.

Wexler, N. S. & Young, A. B. et al. (1987). "Homozygotes for Huntington's disease." *Nature. 326(6109)*, 194-7.

Wheeler, V. C. & White, J. K. et al. (2000). "Long glutamine tracts cause nuclear localization of a novel form of huntingtin in medium spiny striatal neurons in HdhQ92 and HdhQ111 knock-in mice." *Hum. Mol. Genet. 9(4)*, 503-13.

Wheeler, V. C. & Gutekunst, C. A. et al., (2002). "Early phenotypes that presage late-onset neurodegenerative disease allow testing of modifiers in Hdh CAG knock-in mice". *Hum. Mol. Genet.*, 11,633-40.

Yu, Z. X. & Li , S. H. et al. (2003). "Mutant huntingtin causes context-dependent neurodegeneration in mice with Huntington's disease." *J. Neurosci. 23(6)*, 2193-202.

Zala, D. & Colin, E. et al., (2008). "Phosphorylation of mutant huntingtin at S421 restores anterograde and retrograde transport in neurons". *Hum. Mol. Genet.*, *15*, 17(24), 3837-46

Zeitlin, S. & Liu J. P. et al. (1995). "Increased apoptosis and early embryonic lethality in mice nullizygous for the Huntington's disease gene homologue." *Nat. Genet. 11(2)*, 155-63.

Zeron, M. M. & Hansson, O. et al. (2002). "Increased sensitivity to N-methyl-D-aspartate receptor-mediated excitotoxicity in a mouse model of Huntington's disease." *Neuron. 33(6)*, 849-60.

Zhou, H. & Cao, F. et al. (2003). "Huntingtin forms toxic NH2-terminal fragment complexes that are promoted by the age-dependent decrease in proteasome activity." *J. Cell Biol. 163(1)*, 109-18.

Zoghbi, H. Y. & Orr, H. T. (2000). "Glutamine repeats and neurodegeneration." *Annu. Rev. Neurosci. 23*, 217-47.

Zoghbi, H. Y. & Orr, H. T. (2009). "Pathogenic mechanisms of a polyglutamine-mediated neurodegenerative disease, spinocerebellar ataxia type 1". *J. Biol. Chem. 284(12)*,7425-9.

INDEX

A

acid, 23, 36, 42, 43
ADP, 35
adulthood, 2
age, vii, 2, 3, 4, 6, 11, 12, 13, 14, 15, 17, 23, 40, 47, 50
aggregates, 4, 22, 27, 28, 29, 30, 32, 42, 43, 44, 47, 49
aggregation, vii, 22, 46
alanine, 2
allele, 3, 18
amino acids, 23, 24, 28
amygdala, 26
androgen, 30
anger, 6
apoptosis, 35, 44, 47, 49, 50
arrest, 48
aspartate, 15, 49, 50
astrogliosis, 26
asymptomatic, 16
ataxia, 7, 23, 50
ATP, 15, 35
atrophy, 7, 14, 19, 20, 23, 26, 31, 44, 46
authors, 13, 18
autopsy, 18
autosomal dominant, 4
axonal degeneration, 27, 44
axons, 26, 27, 33

B

basal ganglia, 6, 20
base pair, 16
behavior, 2, 33, 40, 48
bias, 1
binding, 30, 32, 43, 45, 49
bioenergy, 15
birth, 2
births, 10
blindness, 8
body mass index, 13
brain, 15, 20, 21, 24, 25, 26, 28, 29, 30, 33, 34, 40, 41, 42, 43, 44, 45, 47

C

Ca^{2+}, 49
calcium, viii, 35, 46, 49
capsule, 26
cardiomyopathy, 7
Caspase-8, 47
Caucasian population, 10
Caucasians, 10
cDNA, 47
cell, viii, 4, 20, 22, 25, 26, 32, 34, 35, 37, 41, 42, 43, 45, 47
cell death, 4, 37, 43, 47
cell line, 35, 42

cell lines, 35, 42
cell signaling, 34
cerebellum, 20, 26
cerebral cortex, 20, 21
CGC, 7
chaperones, 29
chemotherapy, 41
childhood, 2
children, 2, 4
chorea, vii, 4, 10, 11
choreoathetosis, 8
chromosome, 9, 16, 46
clarity, 4
classification, 49
cleavage, vii, 28, 29, 30, 49, 50
cleavages, 29
clinical presentation, 11, 14
clone, 16
CNS, vii, 15
coding, vii, 3, 5, 23
cognitive deficit, 8, 13, 14, 20
cognitive deficits, 8, 13, 14, 20
cognitive dysfunction, 14
cognitive flexibility, 13
cognitive function, 14
cognitive impairment, 6, 8
cohesins, 46
community, 1
composition, 40
compounds, 39
concordance, 21, 25
conduction, 7
confidence, 12
confidence interval, 12
Congress, iv
connective tissue, 7
control, 27, 33
Copyright, iv
corepressor, 43
correlation, 3, 11, 15, 17, 47
correlations, 10, 14
cortex, vii, 20, 21, 22, 25, 26
cytochrome, 35
cytoplasm, viii, 22, 27, 29, 32
cytoskeleton, 33

D

daily living, 11
damages, iv
dance, 10
database, 39
death, 6, 28, 39, 40, 43, 44, 47
defects, 7, 16, 35, 46
deficit, 35
degenerate, 20
degradation, 19
dementia, 7, 8, 14
dendrites, 27
density, 20, 26, 49
depolarization, 35
depression, 6
detection, 18
developmental disorder, 2
diabetes, 7
directionality, 34
disease gene, 4, 41, 42, 43, 46, 48, 50
disease progression, 2, 13, 14, 15, 27, 30, 46
diseases, 3, 4, 10, 19, 27, 39, 48
disequilibrium, 9, 16
disorder, 10, 14, 16
dissociation, 33
distribution, vii, 26, 45
DNA, vii, 9, 16, 17, 23, 26, 32, 42
dominance, 16
Drosophila, 31, 33, 42, 48
duplication, 2
duration, 15
dystonia, 8, 11

E

elderly, 17
encoding, 2
energy, 35, 36, 43, 44, 48
epidemiology, 39, 42
epilepsy, 48
ethnic groups, 10
excitotoxicity, 26, 50
expressivity, 1, 2

eye movement, 11

F

facial muscles, 10
failure, 8
family, 49
FDA, 31
fertility, 8
fibers, 15
fragments, 22, 28, 29, 30, 43, 44, 47
frontal cortex, 21
fusion, 42

G

gait, 10, 11
gene, vii, 3, 9, 10, 15, 16, 17, 21, 22, 23, 24, 25, 26, 27, 28, 29, 30, 31, 32, 34, 35, 36, 40, 43, 45, 47, 49
gene expression, 15, 21, 22, 30, 31, 36, 43, 45
gene promoter, 27
generation, 17, 25, 30
genes, 2, 16, 23, 30, 32, 43
genetic counselling, 19
genetic defect, vii, 23
genetic factors, 13
genetic linkage, 9, 16
genetic marker, 16
genetics, 1, 2, 4
genotype, 17
glia, viii, 26
globus, 20, 26
glutamate, 26, 46
grades, 20, 26
grading, 21
gray matter, 14
growth, 32, 44, 48
growth factor, 32, 44, 48
gynecomastia, 8

H

haplotypes, 16, 45
heterogeneity, 40
hippocampus, 20, 25, 30
histone, 31, 42
hybrid, 32
hybridization, 21
hypothalamus, 26, 33
hypothesis, 25, 28, 31, 32, 36

I

ideal, 16
identification, 25
in situ hybridization, 21
in vitro, 35
in vivo, 15, 27, 32, 44, 48
inclusion, 4, 39, 40
inheritance, 4, 16
inherited disorder, 39
inhibition, 31, 36, 41
inhibitor, 42
injury, iv, 26
inositol, 32, 49
insertion, 2
instability, 2, 18, 43, 47
insulin, 7
insulin resistance, 7
interaction, viii, 33, 35, 42
interactions, vii, viii, 4, 30, 32, 33, 41, 44
interference, 34
interneurons, 20, 26
interval, 12
ion channels, 46
isolation, 29

K

killing, 4

L

language, 13
lesions, 48
life expectancy, 18
life span, 28
likelihood, 40
linkage, 9, 16
localization, viii, 9, 19, 27, 30, 42, 44, 46, 50
locus, 40, 48
lymphoblast, 35

M

machinery, 19
magnetic resonance, 20
magnetic resonance imaging, 20
majority, 17, 29
management, 36
mapping, 9, 16
measures, 15
membranes, 43
memory, 14
mental retardation, 2, 3, 7, 48
mental state, 20
metabolism, 25, 33, 43, 44, 48
mice, 15, 22, 24, 25, 26, 27, 28, 29, 32, 35, 40, 41, 44, 45, 47, 48, 49, 50
microscopy, 22
mitochondria, 35, 36
model, 11, 15, 25, 29, 30, 31, 34, 40, 41, 42, 44, 45, 46, 49, 50
models, vii, 25, 26, 27, 28, 30, 31, 37, 39, 40
monozygotic twins, 13, 48
mood, 11, 14
morphometric, 20, 46, 47
mortality, 40
mothers, 13
motif, 49
motor control, 14
movement, 10, 11
MRI, 14, 20, 47

mRNA, 22, 24
muscular dystrophy, 2, 40
mutant, vii, viii, 19, 25, 26, 27, 28, 29, 30, 31, 32, 33, 34, 35, 36, 37, 39, 41, 42, 43, 44, 45, 47, 49, 50
mutation, vii, 1, 2, 3, 7, 9, 16, 17, 25, 36, 40, 45

N

neocortex, 20
nerve, 33
nerve growth factor, 33
neurodegeneration, vii, 3, 20, 25, 28, 30, 31, 37, 41, 42, 45, 48, 50
neurodegenerative diseases, vii, 3, 23, 35, 48
neurodegenerative disorders, 2
neurogenesis, 37
neurons, viii, 20, 26, 29, 30, 33, 35, 36, 37, 40, 41, 44, 45, 49, 50
neuropsychological tests, 15
neurotoxicity, 19, 29, 33
New England, 12
nuclei, 26, 30
nucleus, viii, 19, 20, 22, 26, 27, 29, 30, 32, 42, 43, 46, 47

O

observations, 14, 17, 25, 31
order, 20
organelles, 25
overload, 35

P

parallel, 45
parameters, 14, 15
parents, 2, 4
parkinsonism, 8
parvalbumin, 26
pathogenesis, 7, 15, 19, 29, 31, 32, 33, 34, 37, 41, 44

pathology, viii, 4, 19, 20, 23, 26, 27, 29, 33, 44, 47
pathways, viii, 32, 34, 37
PCR, 17
penetrance, 1, 2, 4, 10, 16, 18, 45
peptides, 29
performance, 14
peripheral nervous system, vii
permission, iv
personal communication, 18
personality, 6
personality disorder, 6
phenomenology, 18
phenotype, vii, 10, 17, 25, 30, 41, 42, 49
pheochromocytoma, 48
phosphorylation, 15, 34, 40
planning, 15
polymorphism, 47
population, 10, 16
prefrontal cortex, 46
prevention, 30
problem solving, 13, 15
production, vii, 35
progressive neurodegenerative disorder, vii, 6
project, 20
promoter, 27
properties, 31
protective role, vii
protein misfolding, 27
protein structure, 3
protein-protein interactions, 34, 37
proteins, vii, viii, 4, 22, 23, 24, 25, 26, 29, 30, 32, 33, 42, 43, 45
proteolysis, 28, 29, 30, 43

Q

quality control, 19

R

range, vii, 3, 12, 14, 17, 18
recall, 14

receptors, 32, 49
recognition, 1, 14
recombination, 9, 16
recommendations, iv
reconstruction, 21
refining, 16
reflexes, 8
region, 9, 16, 29, 30, 45, 47
regulation, 37, 46
relationship, 11, 12, 13, 14, 35, 39, 42
relatives, 17
relevance, 17, 31
remission, 6
residues, 23
respect, 37
restriction fragment length polymorphis, 16
retardation, 7
retinopathy, 8
ribonucleic acid, 34
rights, iv
risk, 10, 16, 17, 19, 39, 45
RNA, 3, 7, 8, 34
RNA processing, 3

S

scavengers, 15
schizophrenia, 47
search, 9, 32
segregation, 24
selectivity, 15
sensitivity, 50
sensitization, 49
serine, 33, 34
severity, 11, 14, 20, 47
sex, 11, 13
sharing, 2
short-term memory, 13
siblings, 10, 16
signaling pathway, 32
skeletal muscle, 15, 44, 48
sodium, 41
spasticity, 8
species, 23
spectrum, 2

speech, 8, 11
starvation, 36
stimulus, 15
strategies, 13, 16, 37, 39
strategy, 22, 34
striatum, vii, 15, 20, 21, 22, 25, 26, 30
structural changes, 14
Sun, 30, 49
suppression, 3
survival, 41
susceptibility, 36
symptom, 14
symptoms, 10, 14, 16, 18, 20, 25, 28, 37
synaptic plasticity, 37
synaptic transmission, 43
synaptic vesicles, 33
syndrome, 1, 2, 3, 49
synthesis, 15

T

targets, 37
TBP, 8, 31
tenants, 4
terminals, 33
testing, 17, 18, 47, 50
therapeutic interventions, 13, 37
therapeutic targets, viii
therapeutics, 36, 40
therapy, 39
threshold, 3, 4, 43
tissue, 43
toxic effect, 22
toxicity, vii, 19, 25, 27, 29, 42, 44, 46
transcription, 25, 30, 31, 32, 34, 43, 46, 48, 49
transcription factors, 30, 31, 49
transgene, 37
transition, 15
translocation, 29
transmission, 1, 4, 13
transport, 22, 24, 25, 32, 33, 34, 40, 41, 42, 50
tremor, 7, 8
tyrosine, 44

U

uniform, 11

V

variability, 2
variance, 11
variations, 20
vesicle, viii, 33
vulnerability, 20, 21

W

weakness, 7, 8
weight loss, 13

Y

YAC, 27, 42
yeast, 32